HOW TO GET DRESSED

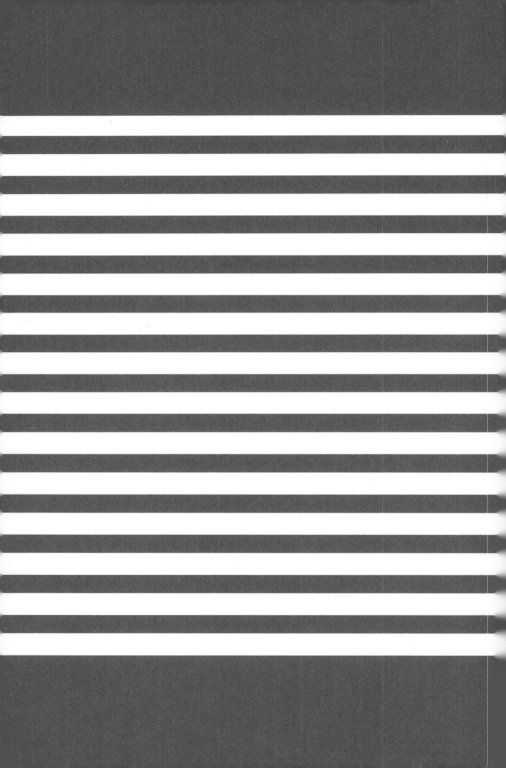

HOW TO GET
DRESSED

A Costume Designer's Secrets for Making Your
Clothes Look, Fit, and Feel Amazing

BY
ALISON FREER

Illustrations by Julia Kuo

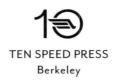

TEN SPEED PRESS
Berkeley

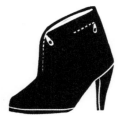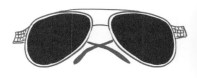

contents

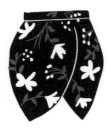 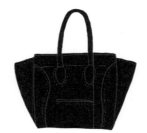 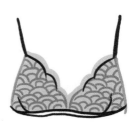

Introduction: Good Clothes Open All Doors

I am a costume designer living and working in Hollywood, California. You might be wondering what a costume designer even does, which makes sense—I wondered the same thing, even as I was agreeing to be one! If you've ever thought that your favorite character's wardrobe on that really great show was the bee's knees, you have a costume designer to thank for it. Because that character didn't just wake up that way—a clever costume designer created the look you love so much.

Being a costume designer means I'm the one responsible for the designing, fabricating, shopping, fitting, accessorizing, altering, repairing, and customizing of every single piece of clothing that actors wear while on camera—right down to their underwear and socks. Whether I'm working on a film, TV show, or commercial, I'm pounding the pavement at fabric stores, boutiques, flea markets, shopping malls, and costume houses twelve to fourteen hours a day, every day. The jobs I take are particularly unglam—because there is a world of difference between a professional costume designer who dresses actors as the characters they play and a celebrity stylist who exclusively outfits stars for red carpet appearances.

One of us (the celebrity stylist) has every top clothing and jewelry designer in the world on speed dial, while the other (the costume designer, that's me!) usually has only five hundred bucks and a pocket full of ingenuity to get the job done. You're not likely to find me delivering ball gowns to hotel suites in glamorous locales or being namechecked in an actor's Oscar acceptance speech. More often than not, I'm standing on a ladder in a dusty costume house looking for showgirl outfits or hunched over a folding table in my basement office on a studio lot, trying to figure out how to sew soda cans onto a furry seal costume in time for the afternoon's shoot. But I wouldn't have it any other way, because the thousands of hours I've spent in the trenches figuring out what works for my actors' wardrobes has made me an authority on anything and everything having to do with clothes—from determining what constitutes proper fit to what to do when a wardrobe crisis strikes. I've also made a ton of mistakes along the way, so whatever your particular problem, I can guarantee it's happened to me—and that I probably have the solution.

I actually lied my way into becoming a costume designer. (That's some hot career advice right there, by the way: fake it 'til you make it!) I've been a rabid collector of clothes, shoes, handbags, and accessories my entire life—so much so that my first apartment in Los Angeles really just functioned as one giant closet. There were rhinestone cowboy boots lining the walls of my living room, a dozen cut-up vintage prom dresses hanging in the bathroom, and nothing in my bedroom but racks of clothes and a mattress on the floor. One day my neighbor (who also happened to be a commercial director) came over to borrow something, took one look at this total mania, and asked, "Whoa, are you a costume designer?"

He didn't even notice the white polyester dress I had bubbling away in a pot on the stove, which was an unsuccessful attempt to dye it black using India ink. (There aren't enough words to explain how badly that experiment failed, by the way—so save yourself a headache and skip to chapter 10 for some pro-style dyeing tips if you're interested in making the things you own change colors.) I froze for all of three seconds before I decided to answer that yes, of course, I was indeed a costume designer. I suspected that whatever a costume designer actually was, I could probably be one. I innately knew that what I already loved doing could probably become my career and that I likely could be just as good at it as anybody else. That director called to hire me for a small commercial the very next week. And just like that, my career was born. It wasn't fate, it was just an incredible opportunity that I smartly grabbed—and then held on to for dear life.

People always ask me what special skills I learned to become a successful costume designer and are consistently shocked when I tell them that the answer is "Pretty much none!" Not only did I not attend fashion school, I barely attended college. I struck out on my own early in life, taking on a number of jobs that depended solely on my ability to communicate well and get people excited about things. I was a shopgirl in clothing and jewelry stores, and the experience I gained while working with the general public is what most effectively prepared me to be a costume designer—because dressing people is really all about sales. I can paint a picture with words and images that allows people to believe in me and see what the end result will be—and give them the confidence to let me spend rather large amounts of their money!

Long before I worked retail, I was a scrappy eighteen-year-old DJ at my local alternative radio station. I started out as the receptionist but eventually badgered them until they broke down and gave me an overnight on-air shift, provided it didn't interfere with my daytime responsibilities. I slept in my office (which was also the station's front lobby) from the time my shift ended at 5:00 a.m. until my daytime receptionist gig began at 9:00 a.m. I learned how to talk, communicate, schmooze, and how to "figure it out" at all costs—skills I'm still utilizing to this very day.

That's not to say that I don't still wake up almost every single morning wondering, "Why do these people trust me? What's wrong with them? And what if I screw everything up?" I've learned the hard way not to psych myself out too much—to just push through and focus solely on the task at hand. This single-minded, eyes-on-the prize, dogged determination is what makes me uniquely qualified to solve any wardrobe problem the universe manages to come up with. (It's also the reason I can't ever attend a wedding without being grabbed out of the congregation at the last minute to tie the bride's French bustle or repair a flapping bra strap.)

Looking back, I'd really been preparing to become a costume designer my entire life—I just never realized it. As a teen in Texas, I'd be dropped off at the mall by my parents each and every Saturday with my five best buds and $30 of babysitting money in my pocket. While my pals were busy blowing their allowance on CDs and Slurpees, I was hunting for cool clothes I could actually afford that fit the vision of myself I had in my head. (Figuring out what image I wanted to project to the world via my wardrobe makes me the very first character I ever dressed!) This was a valuable lesson—because while having great style is an essential part of being a costume designer, good budgeting skills are really at the heart of the job description. Designers who go over budget don't tend to get rehired, so knowing your way around a clearance rack is a very valuable skill.

Being a costume designer means that when things go wrong, I'm the one who takes the heat. You haven't really lived until you've gotten a shocking amount of red lipstick out of a white Gucci blouse in front of a live studio audience because someone hugged an actor too force-fully in the middle of a taping. It costs about $1,000 per minute while the camera is held and everyone waits for me to fix it. Situations like that are why I've had to come up with a stable of solutions to disasters that really work—and work incredibly fast. Wardrobe disasters are a way of life when you're a costume designer, and I've had every single one possible happen to me at some point in my career. So the next time you find yourself suffering from a terrible clothing malfunction, you can take heart in knowing that what you are experiencing has likely happened to your favorite star as well. But you can also rest easy—because now that you're holding this book, you've got the solu-tion to almost any dastardly wardrobe disaster that could occur.

In the coming pages, I'm going to pull back the curtain and show you what really goes on behind the scenes at a wardrobe fitting. We'll figure out together who the heck you really are and what your clothes are saying about you, and I'll let you in on all the style secrets my actors probably wish I wouldn't—while teaching you how to keep the clothes you've already got in your closet in tip-top shape. (Because, yes, wardrobes need tune-ups and maintenance, too.) I'll also open up my costume designer's tool kit and share all the gadgets I use to make those stars look like stars. Because the old saying really is true: Good clothes open all doors. But I'm of the belief that it's not so much *what* you wear that makes people sit up and take notice—it's how you wear it. By the time you're done reading here, there won't be a single one of my secrets you won't know. Everyone's wardrobe could benefit from having a professional costume designer (and her secret bag of tricks) in their back pocket—and that's just what this book is: Me, Alison Freer, at your service.

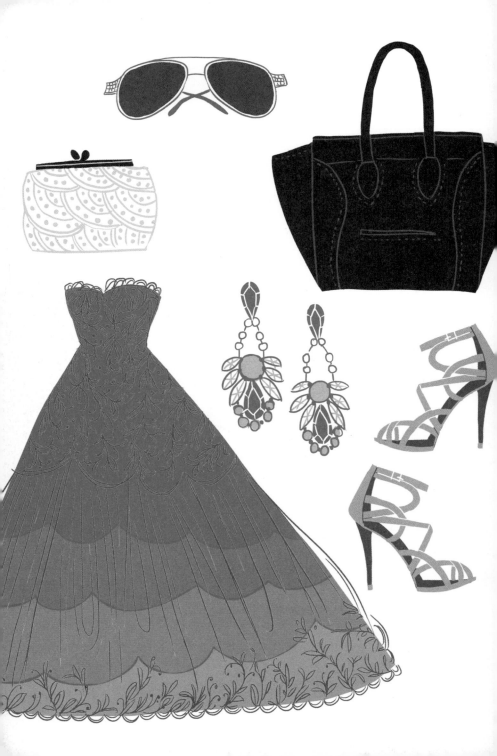

CHAPTER
1

MOVIE MAGIC:
or, why movie stars look like movie stars

Imagine walking into a room bathed in warm light with flattering mirrors all around. Racks and racks of clothes stand before you, all in your exact size. Rows of beautiful shoes are lined up on the floor like good little soldiers. Tray after tray of sparkling accessories and jewelry are nearby. And just for good measure, there is a small selection of bras and a few terrifyingly unidentifiable underthings at the ready.

If you ever find yourself in this situation, congrats! You are a Hollywood actor at a luxurious wardrobe fitting. (If you are a really big deal, a production assistant will be standing by to take your coffee or lunch order.) Sounds awesome, right? It is, except now you have to take off all your clothes in front of the costume designer, her assistant, and a tailor—then stand still while they pin, poke, and pout at an endless parade of clothes on your body. The final result will be total on-camera perfection, but let's back up and talk about how that room full of clothes got there in the first place. All those clothes don't just magically appear at a fitting, despite what producers in Hollywood might think.

Where you begin the journey to a successful wardrobe fitting really depends on what you happen to be shooting—a commercial, film, music video, or TV show. Each project has a very specific set of needs, and the only constant in the life of a costume designer is that those needs will change on a dime. The needs of a single project could take you all the way from a shop in Chinatown, begging the proprietor to have her cousin bring over fifty more pairs of ninja shoes from their warehouse in time for your fitting at noon, and spit you out at a pet store, trying to determine which of the thirteen dog tuxedos they carry can be altered to fit a turtle. (Yes, the ninja shoes and the turtle tux were indeed for the same shoot. Ain't Hollywood grand?)

FIRST, YOU HAVE TO PREPARE

Let's use a TV show as an example. My first order of business is to read the script carefully and flesh out each character's backstory.

When the script says "Heather, twenty-five years old, perpetually single," it's up to me to fill in the blanks, both through my imagination and via many detailed conversations with the show's creator—often called the executive producer or EP. On a film, the costume designer works hand-in-hand with the director to determine each charcter's look. On a commercial, you've got to sift through a mountain of differing ideas, opinions, and notes from the director, client, agency, and producer—all before you get to start designing anything. But let's get back to our TV script—where does this perpetually single Heather work? How much money does she make? Where does she like to shop? What kind of music does she listen to? What books does she read over and over? These are the questions I have to ask before I ever even step foot in a store to shop, as the answers greatly inform a character's style.

Once I've filled in the blanks, I begin the most fun part of my job—making look books. A look book is a visual reference of each character's style touchstones. To make one, I utilize online images, tear sheets from magazines, photos I've snapped while walking around town, and various film, music, and book references. This process involves a ton of back and forth with my bosses—including hundreds of phone calls and a quantity of emails that nobody besides a stalker should be sending to another human being. But at this point in the process, excessive communication is key. Nailing the character's look via a visual presentation is a tool that will serve us throughout the entire production. A good look book is a filter to run every wardrobe decision through, and it's the reason that halfway through a show, I can look at a garment on the rack and tell immediately if it's right for the character or not.

With that hurdle cleared, I shift into practical mode. I take a second look at the script (which has most likely undergone a rewrite by this point) and break it down according to how many story days there are, what each character's specific wardrobe needs are, and if any actor has a gag that involves multiple sets of the exact same outfit. When you need three sets of an outfit on a TV show, it's most likely because something really bad is going to happen to it. Sitcoms in particular are obsessed with squirting anything viscous in actors' faces—and the grosser, the better! Oil, (fake) blood, mashed potatoes, and mayonnaise are perennial favorites. Now you are seeing the whole picture: being an actor is not quite as glam as you might think. Which reminds me: Have you ever wondered what's really in that freaky green slime used on a certain famous kids' network? The formula varies ever so slightly each time it's mixed, but it usually involves a truly disgusting combination of vanilla pudding and green food coloring mixed with applesauce, oatmeal, and baby shampoo. (The baby shampoo is meant to make it easier to wash out of the actor's hair, but it really only helps so much.)

Once I have a clear idea of what's needed, I have a big meeting with my entire costume crew, which usually averages between five and seven people. This crew includes my right hand, the show's costume supervisor. The costume supervisor is responsible for a little bit of everything that goes on in our department—from shopping for clothes and scheduling labor to planning fittings, paying the bills, dressing background actors, and performing emergency alterations. We also have a costume illustrator who works with me to help design all our custom-made pieces, plus two full-time, dedicated shoppers who hit the malls, costume houses, boutiques, and thrift stores every single day in an endless cycle of shopping for stuff we need and returning what's been rejected. (When store clerks see us coming, they usually run the other way!) Our standby tailor (who can make, alter, or tailor absolutely anything) rounds out our crew, along with our set costumer—the person responsible for keeping track of who wore what when. TV shows are shot completely out of order—and it's not uncommon to film small parts of one simple scene in tiny bits over the course of five or more days. So forgetting if an actor had his tie tied or not would result in it jumping from done to undone in the middle of a scene. Our set costumer keeps everything straight by taking copious photos of the actors in their costumes and writing pages of detailed notes in our "bible"—also known as the wardrobe continuity book. That way, there's no possibility of making an error.

The set costumer is like the paparazzi of the wardrobe department—grabbing actors for stealth photos anywhere they can. Certain actors hate having their picture taken, so we are sometimes reduced to grabbing photos on the sly so they don't realize what we were doing. This stealth photography results in some hilariously terrible photos of the world's most beautiful people. Stars: They're just like us!

Together, my costume crew and I pore over each character's look book and brainstorm spots to shop, get any specialty custom-made pieces we need in the works, and come up with a color palette to suit the actor that has now been cast in each role. There are a lot of differing opinions to service on a show, from the director who only likes blue to the actor who refuses to wear a skirt—even though her character is described as a miniskirt-wearing sexpot. It's like a puzzle, made all the more exciting by the fact that we usually have less than twenty-four hours to prepare for each actor's fitting.

IT'S TIME TO SHOP

Once we have a plan, it's time to hit the stores. Shopping for a production is always a mad, hectic dash to find the specific items we need in a very short amount of time. (And includes an amount of mania over socks you'd have to see to believe.) I once had to have my mom frantically overnight me twelve pairs of red lifeguard trunks from a store near her house in Texas when I couldn't get my hands on any locally, only to find out ten minutes after she shipped them that the whole scene we needed them for had been cut. It's like an epic scavenger hunt, full of thrilling victories and agonizing defeats.

The whole shopping process is made even more exciting by the fact that we are forever shooting a Christmas episode in July or doing a beach-themed show in the dead of winter, when no store has a tank top or a single, solitary swimsuit to save my miserable life. If we start to strike out at all our usual spots, I send someone back to the office pronto to start some serious research—calling each and every store we can think of until we finally find that needle in the haystack. This includes, but is not limited to, begging salespeople to check their back stock, "Just one more time for me, pretty please?" and calling every acquaintance you happen to have in your phone, asking if they've seen polka-dotted skirts for sale anywhere recently.

When we really can't find what we need in stores or online, I head straight to the fabric store to grab material and have our tailor magically run up exactly what we need, right to order. I will never get over the awe I feel at seeing a lowly bolt of fabric become a beautiful, functioning garment. My own sewing skills are actually somewhat limited—I can repair just about anything and hem a pair of pants in no time. But past that, it would take me a week to whip up a garment that takes my tailor about three hours to make.

Once we've procured everything we could possibly need (or want) for an actor's fitting, we haul it back to the office and set it all up. I organize the racks and preassemble possible outfits according to the script requirements. Shoes get taken out of boxes and lined up neatly on the floor for easy access during the fitting. Every shirt is unbuttoned, ready to be slipped on instantly. An actor's time with us is always limited: if we're very lucky, we get about an hour to figure out twelve or more outfits for an entire show. But in most cases, we get a measly thirty minutes—so every second saved counts. If the lighting and general vibe in the room we've been assigned isn't up to snuff, I drag every lamp, scarf, and candle I own into the office to create a warm, welcoming, dreamy environment. It's part romantic boudoir, part grandma's closet, and part hippie love den.

LET'S HAVE A FITTING

A wardrobe fitting is actually a rather awkward experience. Within two minutes of meeting, I'm asking these actors to shed their clothes and put themselves completely in my hands. It's an enormous amount of trust to ask for right off the bat! This is where my old-school Southern manners come in handy. I always make sure my actors have something to drink, a snack if they want it, a comfortable place to sit, and a spot to hang their coat. Just like in real life, these simple niceties go a long way toward putting nervous actors at ease, making them more likely to enjoy themselves and be receptive to my ideas. The outdated image of a stern wardrobe mistress frowning at an actor who can't fit into a pair of pants is long gone. I am a true sartorial support system, encouraging good feelings and pointing out the design flaws in garments when they don't fit correctly. (I also make sure to have a wide range of sizes on the rack, as nothing sinks a fitting faster than clothes that don't fit.)

If I've done my job correctly, the actors I dress will be able to leave the details of their look to me and are free to concentrate on their lines, their performance, and the director's notes. Getting an actor to trust you is the hardest (yet most rewarding) part of my job. A truly great costume designer is equal parts mind reader, fashionista, and psychotherapist—not to mention good with kids and animals. Dressing people for a living gives you access to their innermost secrets, and it's not something I take lightly.

A successful wardrobe fitting is a slightly chaotic, funny mess. There are clothes flying and jokes being made. Sometimes we take pictures of the worst possible outfits just because they make us laugh so much. I always consider it a coup when I convince actors to try on something they normally wouldn't like and they wind up loving it. This is a big reason why actors tend to look more "fashionable" than us mortals—they have people like me pressing, prodding, and encouraging them to try new things. (It's always good to have someone to encourage you to branch out a bit, style-wise—be it a friend, a salesperson, or a page in a magazine. Having good style is all about taking a risk now and then.)

Once we agree on the best looks from our fitting and the tailor has pinned the pieces that need alterations, I photograph the actor in everything and submit the photos to the powers that be for approval. I then have one final "check fit" with the actor to iron out any last-minute details. When everyone involved finally agrees that everything looks good, we are locked and loaded—and ready to shoot!

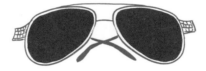

HOW DO THEY MAKE A TV SHOW, ANYWAY?

The shooting process for a TV show takes anywhere from two to five days per episode. During that time, my job shifts from costume designer to quality-control technician. When an actor is about to appear on camera in an outfit for the first time, I am on standby outside the dressing room, putting out any last-minute fires. And there are always fires—actors are forever exclaiming at the very last second, "Wait! This doesn't fit! I can't wear it! I suddenly hate it!" This is why I always have a backup look on hand, budget be damned.

I'm also constantly on the move while a show is shooting—doing rounds between my office, the stage, and the director of photography's bay of monitors, keeping an ear out for what my bosses are saying and making sure that what looks good to my naked eye comes across on camera. Watching my work on screen is the number one way I've improved and polished my costuming skills throughout the years. (You can do the same thing at home simply by photographing your outfits and seeing what worked—and what you can adjust next time you wear a particular ensemble.) On an extended series, I'm also usually jumping ahead to the next episode at the same time we're shooting the current one, brainstorming ideas and sourcing whatever weird things the writers have managed to dream up, which could be anything from a bush outfit (made entirely out of sticks and leaves we picked up off the ground) to a realistic taco costume, complete with fabric cheese and lettuce framing the actor's face.

While we are busy shooting, our shoppers shift into return mode. Every unused item is accounted for and taken back to the store it came from. A successful return mission also includes shopping for pieces we need for the following week's episode. (We don't have the luxury of totally closing out our current work before we jump ahead.) It's a real game of mental hopscotch to keep everything straight in my mind. I need to have already read the next script and have an idea of what to tell our shoppers to look for—otherwise they will just sit around, wasting precious prep time. (And I have to do all this while still paying close attention to the script we are currently shooting on stage.) I'd call it a grind, but that wouldn't even come close to describing it. We then lather, rinse, and repeat this process, twelve hours a day, every single day of the week. It's exhausting, but I love it. It's the one thing I'm really good at, where I always have an answer to every single problem—or definitively know when all hope is lost. It's my own special brand of witchcraft. So now you know exactly why those movie stars look like movie stars—and it's due to a lot of behind-the-scenes magic, courtesy of the show's costume department.

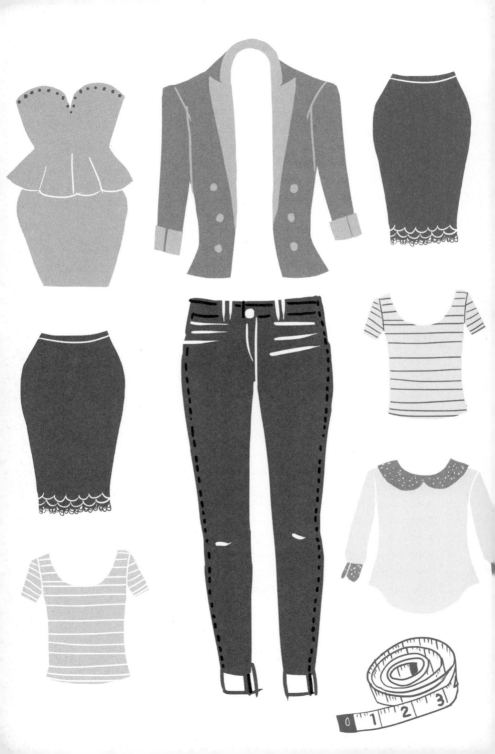

CHAPTER 2

FIT:
the true enemy of great style

Do you ever wonder what people really mean when they say someone has "great style"? It's an elusive concept, to be sure. What they are really saying is that the person in question just looks good all the time, but when pressed to explain, most folks would have a hard time putting their finger on exactly what it is about that person's look that makes it seem so effortless. Well, let me tell you a secret: the reason you think that some people have such good style is simply because they always wear clothes that fit them—and fit them well. When you banish ill-fitting clothes from your life and only allow proper fitting ones in, you open the door to having great style—forever.

It's a total lie that you need a certain body type to be truly stylish. Style is not something you're just born with or tough luck to you, kitten. Being fashionable doesn't mean a lifetime of shoes that kill, fretting that something is "so last season," or waiting to wear something "as soon as I lose five pounds." And skinny isn't a goal—it's a style of jean. The real, true enemy of great style is fit. Because if your clothes don't fit you properly, you'll never look amazing. Once you learn how to tell if a garment is fitting you as it's supposed to, you'll be amazed at how much better you look and feel in your clothes. But *fit* is a loaded word—and it should come as no surprise to you that the Hollywood definition of it is actually a total lie.

When I dress an actor for a photo, I go to great lengths to make their garments appear to fit them perfectly. But notice I said "appear"—because while that outfit you see a celeb wearing in a magazine may look flawless from the front, you'd be mighty surprised if you saw what was probably going on in the back. It's usually a crazy jumbled mess of pins, clamps, and double-stick tape holding it all together, faking a perfect fit—which is not something that would ever work in real life.

Fit is actually a fairly clinical, mechanical concept. It refers to the garment needing to be right for the body, not the body somehow being wrong for the garment. And the idea of fit gets way stickier when you start to hold it up to the light and examine it a bit more closely—because while it really is merely a function of how a garment is performing, it's also highly subjective. Most guides to proper fit worry about what is or is not "flattering" to your particular body shape or figure. But they all fall short of actually providing any useful information to the reader —because they don't take actual, factual fit into account.

Proper fit means that the clothes you wear should always perform as you need them to, period. That means no garments that gape or bunch, no seams that twist, no pants with crotches that hang too low, no blouses that won't stay buttoned, and no skirts that shift around annoyingly. These everyday nuisances are simply mechanical problems caused by poorly fitting clothes, and they can all be banished in a heartbeat—if you know how your clothes are meant to fit in the first place. Once you learn what the most common fit pitfalls are, you can start to spot and avoid them.

But first things first: you can't even begin to determine if your clothes are fitting properly if you don't have a full-length mirror. Even a $6 one from a discount store leaned up against the wall is miles better than only getting half the picture via your dresser-top mirror. Once you've got that covered, you can move on to banishing bad fit from your life. Because great fit equals great style—always.

THE RIGHT PANTS

Finding a pair of pants that fit correctly is a nightmare for almost every single woman. Take heart—you are not alone! From petite to tall or curvy to stick figure, it's a constant battle to find something in your price range that doesn't pull, tug, ride up, or bunch unflatteringly. And if you happen to be supermodel height? Good luck finding an inseam long enough to graze the top of your shoes. You're likely going to spend the rest of your life pretending that ankle-cropped pants are "so totally *in* right now!"

Let's start by talking about denim. Jeans are one of the hardest pant styles to nail down properly. I regularly bring twenty or more pairs of jeans in for an actor's first fitting—and we end up trying on almost every single one! Maybe you find that that all jeans have a tendency to slip down, exposing your backside and underwear to the world. There's also a high probability that most jeans you've tried on manage to dig into your stomach in an uncomfortable, unsupportive way. These problems often occur when a person with a long torso chooses a style of jean that is cut way too low in the waist, cutting her off right at the middle.

The right tool to solve these problems is a higher-waisted jean— so in the future, you long torso-ed gals will know to seek them out, no matter what style is allegedly "in" that season. Forget boring haters droning on about "mom jeans," because a higher waistline will hit your tummy at a better spot and act like a corset: giving support and providing a long, uninterrupted line when you bend over. (Which also means zero panty flashing!) And since they fit snugly around your actual waist and not low on your hips, they won't slide down every five seconds.

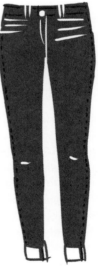

The takeaway here is that when you find something that fits your body and performs the action you want it to, nobody notices whether it's technically "in" or "out." They just think you look great—all the time—and that particular fit then becomes a permanent part of your personal wardrobe toolkit. Knowing what fits you properly takes almost all the confusion out of shopping— instantly. (Insert giant sigh of relief here.)

THE RIGHT PANTS HAVE THE RIGHT RISE
But why does a high-waisted pair of jeans fit those with long torsos better than other styles?

It's all due to the "rise" of a particular pair of pants, also known as the distance between the crotch and the waistband. It's an important detail, because the shorter this length, the lower the pants will sit on your waist. To start figuring out what the best rise is for you, take a flexible cloth tape measure (not a metal one from the hardware store!) and determine the distance from the top of the waistband to the bottom of the crotch seam on your favorite-fitting pair of pants.

A low-rise pair will start a good three inches below the natural waist, so any soft flesh will spill over. But a pair with a higher rise (that's the high-waisted pair we discussed before) will hit you just above your natural waist, holding you in and increasing your physical comfort many times over. If a pair of pants isn't fitting you properly, it's usually due to having chosen the wrong rise measurement for your body. Now I've told you everything I know about pants with a high rise, perfect for those of you with a longer torso, but what about all those other pants out there?

REGULAR OR MID RISE: Regular or mid-rise pants are meant to be worn just below your natural waist, which is found at the point where your waist is narrowest. Some folks think their natural waist is right at the navel, but this is incorrect. Just as no two bodies are alike, everyone's natural waist is at a different spot. Your true natural waist is to be found at the smallest point of your torso. If you seem to have lost your natural waist and need a little help finding it again, just stand up and bend from side to side while nude. The highest point along your midsection where your skin creases and folds is your natural waist. (And take note: Some folks' natural waists are very high—mine is right at the bottom of my ribcage!)

Most pants (such as casual chinos or simple wool trousers) have a regular or mid rise. If you have a somewhat high natural waist (more than an inch above your navel), pants with too low of a rise can cause the center seam to ride up and put the entire outline of your crotch (sometimes uncharitably called a "camel toe") on full display. But a pair with a regular rise will give a more relaxed fit—and alleviate the problem completely. (This particular problem has long been judgingly considered a by-product of wearing pants that are too tight, but it's actually just a simple engineering problem—easily fixable by choosing the right fit.)

LOW RISE: Low-rise pants are meant to be worn at the hips and will sit well below your natural waist—which means roughly two inches or more below your navel. They obviously aren't intended to conform to your natural waist, as the proper fit of a pair of low-rise pants is meant to mimic the "hip-hugger" styles of the 1960s and 1970s. If you have short legs and a long torso, low-rise pants are unlikely to fit you properly.

ULTRALOW RISE: The lowest of the low, a pair of pants with an ultralow rise will start at least four (if not five) inches below the navel, often just barely grazing the bottom of your hipbone. If you are very short-waisted (meaning the distance between your shoulders and your waist is less than most clothes are generally designed for), a pair of ultralow rise pants can be the perfect fit solution to bring your look into proportion.

SHORT RISE: Often found in the petite section, short-rise pants are meant to be worn at the natural waist of a shorter person. A shorter rise means you won't have a bunch of extra material in the crotch— which equals more comfort and a better fit on shorter bodies.

SAY GOODBYE TO POCKETS THAT POP OPEN (AND OTHER ANNOYING PANTS PROBLEMS)

Those of you with more generous hips will find that the pockets on dress pants tend to pop out unflatteringly. The right tool to solve this problem is either a pair of pants that zip along the side seam or have horizontal pockets that simply can't gap or pull—by design.

When we have this problem on shows, we simply have the pockets stitched closed—sometimes removing the pocket lining as well. But this fix is not reserved solely for actors in glamorous Hollywood, California! It's something you can actually have a tailor do quite cheaply—and it's well worth the money. (For the whole scoop on all the little alterations you can have done easily and inexpensively to make your clothes look better, flip ahead to chapter 3!)

Another common fit problem on less expensive pants (although I've seen it on $300 pairs, too) is a poorly set zipper that pulls, gaps, and falls down slowly yet surely—usually while you are right in the middle of talking to someone important. There is absolutely no fix for this besides sewing the zipper shut every single time you wear them, which is a completely ridiculous idea. So always take a brisk lap around the store and vigorously sit down/stand up in the dressing room a few times to ensure the pair you are considering buying does not have any zipper problems that could cause embarrassment later on.

If a pair of pants pull and "whisker" at the crotch or groin area when you try them on, beware—as this is not a problem that can be fixed by any alteration. It doesn't always mean they are too small—more often than not, it just means they are poorly designed. Pants that pull and wrinkle across the very tops of your thighs will cause them to fit poorly everywhere else, too. Getting the proper fit in a pair of pants is a true house of cards—because when one part of the structure is off, the whole thing is doomed! If they aren't sitting properly on your hips, they'll be far more likely to ride up your bum, gap at the waist, and end up being too short—all because they don't fit correctly at that one specific area.

A BETTER SKIRT

A skirt is usually a far easier fit than a pair of pants—but that doesn't mean just any old one will do. A badly made skirt (or one that simply doesn't fit you properly) brings its own set of problems to the table. The main thing my actors complain about when wearing a skirt is the tendency to spin around and shift while walking. This is usually caused

by choosing a skirt that doesn't sit properly at your natural waistline—not your hips, mind you—I'm talking about your actual, factual
waistline, which we found back on page 15.

When a skirt fits properly on your waist, it anchors itself in place
around your waist and hips—and that helps the skirt stay in place all
day long without shifting or twisting. If you have a look at the skirts
in your closet that are guilty of rotating annoyingly around your
body when you walk, you'll likely notice they are cut fairly straight up
and down. This cylindrical shape makes a skirt sit lower on the hips,
allowing it to spin around to its heart's content with every step. This
problem happens most commonly with pencil skirts—and is usually
worse for women with bigger hips; in order to get a proper fit through
the bum and thighs, they're left with a skirt that is too big in the waist,
which means the skirt has no anchor, so round and round and round
it goes. The easy, inexpensive solution to this problem is to simply buy
your skirts in a size that fits you through the hips and thighs correctly—
then have a tailor add darts at the waistband to provide more shape,
keeping the skirt firmly in place.

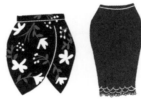

Buying bigger and then taking in only where needed is the costume
designer's ultimate secret weapon for dressing curves—and it really
works! But even women with stick straight or boyish hips are likely to
find they have the exact same skirt-spinning problem. Luckily, it can
also be easily fixed by having a tailor add darts at the waist. Darts

are a truly magical trick for making clothes that are just a bit "off" fit properly—so if you aren't sure what the heck I'm getting at when I talk about them, jump ahead to page 36 to learn more!

Pencil skirts are definitely the hardest style of skirt to get a proper fit in, but other types can present problems as well—so it helps to know a bit about how a few different basic skirt styles are meant to fit in the first place. But keep in mind: As long as a skirt fits like it's supposed to through the waist and hips, the rest of it becomes a simple matter of personal style.

A-LINE: Named for its shape, which resembles a capital letter A. An A-line skirt is typically knee-length, and usually does not feature any embellishments, pleats, or slits. A properly fitted A-line skirt should be wider at the lower hip than at the waist.

CIRCLE: Also known as a skater skirt, this is made in a circular shape that flares out at the hem and does not have any darts, pleats or gathers. A properly fitting circle skirt will fit snugly at the waist and flare out from the body. It's a good choice for those who want a full-skirted look without additional bulk.

MAXI: A long skirt that drapes to the ankle. The right hem length for a maxi skirt is either right at the ankle (for taller babes) or just grazing the floor (for petite ladies).

MINI: A skirt that has a hemline well above the knee. The average mini-skirt measures anywhere from ten to fourteen inches from waist to hem. If you are tall, you'll need a miniskirt that hangs lower on the hips for it to be long enough to cover your bum. Shorter babes can choose styles that hit at the natural waistline, as length doesn't pose such a problem.

WRAP: A wrap skirt is exactly what it sounds like—a simple garment, often made of thin cotton, that wraps around the waist and is secured in place by two ties. You'll know if a wrap skirt isn't fitting correctly, as the front will splay open at the knee. This means the skirt is likely too small. A properly fitting wrap skirt will have enough material to overlap in the front and tie at the side, allowing for more coverage in front.

MIDI: A 1970s inspired, slightly fuller style that hits the wearer at or just below the knees. The classic midi skirt will fall right at the middle of the shin, where the leg starts to thin out.

TULIP: Fitted at the waist, with extra folds of fabric at the front and a hem that closely resembles the inverted petals of a tulip flower. A tulip skirt can be tricky to wear if the folds are not secured at the front—as this will allow the two sides to separate and make walking and sitting somewhat tricky.

If you've ever worn a skirt with a side or back zipper, you've likely encountered the annoying "bump" that makes a zipper bunch out in a lumpy and unflattering way. This can be caused by many things, but the most common problem is a difference in the materials used for the skirt itself and for the tape on either side of the zipper. If the skirt is cotton and the zipper tape is made of polyester, the cotton skirt will shrink a bit upon washing or dry cleaning, causing the polyester zipper tape material to get bunched up and wrinkly. (If this is the cause, the only cure is replacing the zipper with a cotton-taped version—something you can read all about on page 38.)

A bumpy zipper can also result if the manufacturer didn't take the time to properly set the zipper—or simply used the wrong zipper for the garment. While an invisible zipper may look great disappearing into the side seam of a skirt, it's not very practical. A side seam is a major stress point on a skirt, and an invisible zipper is simply too wimpy to stand up to the task. It will always pull, wrinkle, and bunch itself up. A bumpy, wavy zipper on a skirt constitutes a bad fit—so unless you're interested in paying to have it replaced, leave it on the rack.

A BRILLIANT BLOUSE

Do you know how to tell if a blouse or shirt fits you properly? You might be surprised to find that you actually don't, as the ways in which one can fit poorly are endless. Anyone with boobs (generous or small!) will have their own list of fit issues to complain about. Luckily, learning what to look for when you first try on a blouse is likely the answer to all your shirt-fit problems. Start in a well-lit room with a good mirror. Button the front and sleeves of the blouse, but don't tuck it in just yet! We want to give it a once-over to determine if it does indeed fit before we get around to seeing how it will look tucked into your favorite pair of jeans.

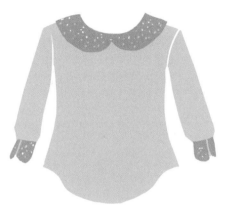

The first thing you'll want to check is the bustline. Big-busted babes will always have a hard time finding a button-front blouse that closes properly and doesn't gap open in between the buttons. You can solve this problem in one of two ways: by either choosing to have a tailor sew tiny snaps in between the buttons to keep your blouse from popping open (this is our go-to fix on set) or by simply swapping out button-front styles for a tunic or popover style blouse and move on with your life, never worrying about gaping buttons again. Removing as many buttons as possible from the equation helps eliminates the problem—and a garment that eliminates problems is the exact definition of proper fit.

If the bustline doesn't gap, pull, or strain at the buttons or seams, you've got the green light to move on to checking out the shoulder fit. To do so, cross your arms over your chest, watching the shoulders of the blouse while you do so. If it bunches at the shoulders, chances are it's too big. Any pulling or tightness at the shoulder indicates the blouse is likely too small. Fixing a poorly fitted shirt shoulder is a complicated alteration that isn't worth doing, so if the next size up or down doesn't solve the problem, don't bother buying it.

If the shoulder fits with no bunching or pulling, congratulations! You're more than halfway there. Next, you'll want to turn your wrists and neck with the blouse completely buttoned. The cuffs and collar should move comfortably without shifting upward or twisting. Make sure you bend over in the blouse (with it both tucked and untucked), checking to see if it rides up too far in the front or back. If it passes the bend test and covers everything you want it to, hooray! There's only one fit issue left to check.

If the blouse has bust darts, you'll want to make sure that they are sitting correctly. Properly placed darts should point toward the bust and end about a half inch away from the nipple; they should never sit above or below the nipple. If the bust darts line up correctly, take a final minute to bend and move in the blouse, checking for any previously unseen pulling or twisting before you finally deem it fit to come live in your closet.

A JACKET FIT FOR A QUEEN

A jacket that fits you well can pull together a look that's seriously lacking in other areas. I keep a tailored jacket in my office on set at all times, as it's the easiest way to make even a t-shirt and jeans seem a bit more polished. But it can't be just any old jacket! As it's usually the cornerstone of an outfit, proper fit is especially important.

The most common fit problem is a jacket that's too snug. If you're going for a very tailored, fitted look, you're more likely to always be toeing the line between too boxy and too tight. This may sound obvious, but if you can't hug somebody without feeling like you're about to bust open a seam, your jacket is too tight. Pulling across your shoulder blades also indicates a too-snug fit. But if you can't button it up easily, you needn't worry. The open jacket look is acceptable in every line of work—unless you happen to be an attorney standing in front of a judge in federal court. If a jacket that closes is high on your wish list, but you can never find one that fits the bill, opt for a structured yet stretchy knit jacket instead. Versions with details such as contrasting buttons or notched collars can stand in for regular suit jackets beautifully—and have the added benefit of stretch, allowing them to actually close over your boobs. (You may have the opposite problem—your jacket fits well in the shoulders but is too big in the waist. If so, flip to page 36 to learn how you can have a tailor add some darts to nip it in at the waist in a jiffy.)

Most jackets have a small amount of padding at the shoulder. This is important, as it gives a jacket its shape. But those pads (and the entire shoulder seam) should stop right at the end of your natural shoulder. If they extend any farther (past your shoulder and down toward your arm), the whole jacket will look too large. Adjusting the shoulder of a jacket is a huge alteration—so you're better off buying one that fits well through the shoulder in the first place.

The sleeve length of your jacket is really a personal choice. While there are no hard and fast rules for women's sleeve lengths as there are for men (more about that on page 202), you can't go wrong with having your jacket cuffs lie somewhere between one inch above the knuckles and one inch below the wrist. I personally like mine a bit shorter (about an inch above the wristbone) to better show off a little more shirt cuff, a sliver of wrist, or a fabulous bracelet!

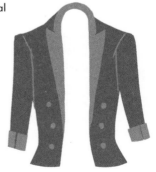

If you have broad shoulders and a small chest, you might find that jackets with lapels tend to sag at the chest area instead of creating a nice, clean vertical line, which in turn causes the jacket to slouch and fit poorly through the entire bust, arm, and shoulder area. This is the very definition of poor fit, but luckily, it's easy enough to fix. Having a tiny snap sewn anywhere from one to two inches above the top button will cause the lapel to lay straighter, better, and flatter—which in turn makes the whole jacket fit better!

THE PERFECT DRESS

The humble dress is quite possibly the world's most perfect garment. The right one can easily be jazzed up or dressed down according to your needs. I put all my female actors in dresses every chance I get. Sometimes the ones who have spent a lifetime wearing only pants will tell me they can't figure out how to perform in a dress. I always remind them that Lucille Ball (of *I Love Lucy* fame) did almost every bit of the show's slapstick comedy while wearing a dress—so why can't they?

But even perfect-looking garments can be bad if they fit poorly. Different dress styles present a variety of fit issues—no matter what your body type. So if you've ever wondered why a certain style just "doesn't work" on you, it's probably due to that particular style's fit limitations. And as you're probably sick of hearing me say by now, it doesn't matter what kind of dress you choose to wear if it doesn't fit correctly! So here's a brief overview of the most common dress styles out there—along with the fit pros and cons of each:

EMPIRE: A dress with an empire seam (one that is sewn directly below the bustline) is a great tool for those with larger breasts, as the design can accommodate a full bust without adding fabric width to the garment's waist and hips. But an empire seam that sits too high on your bust is practically impossible to fix. So if the seam of a dress cuts into the bottom of your boobs, leave it on the rack. Otherwise you'll spend half your life adjusting it until you finally freak out and throw it in the trash in the middle of the day on a Tuesday.

FIT AND FLARE: A style of dress that is narrower at the top, cinched through the waist, and flared through the hips to the hem. A fit and flare dress is a good choice for those with smaller breasts. Unless they are constructed with stretch fabric, fit and flare dresses tend to be too tight at the bust for full-bosomed babes. A fit and flare dress also provides a nice, relaxed fit for those with a generous backside and hips.

SHEATH: A sheath dress is a fitted, straight-cut dress that is often nipped in at the waistline. Usually designed with a structured sleeve, the sheath provides a classic, timeless look—but due to its highly fitted nature can be prone to armhole, shoulder, and waistline fit issues.

+ When the armhole of a sheath dress fits poorly, you'll know it—and the entire dress will then fit poorly. An armhole that is set too high will cause it to dig and cut into your arm and armpit. If an armhole is set too low, the entire dress will pull up when you lift your arms. The armhole on a sheath dress should be no lower than an inch below your armpit to allow for good arm mobility.

+ A well-structured shoulder is the most important feature of a sheath dress. It's the foundation the whole thing is built on! As with a jacket, the shoulder seam should always stop right at the end of your natural shoulder. If it extends past your shoulder and droops down toward your arm, it's not fitting you properly.

+ Be extra careful when purchasing a sheath dress with a very fitted waist; a dress that has a seam in the wrong spot will become uncomfortable very quickly. You'll want the waist seam to hit you right at your natural waist for maximum comfort and optimal fit. As we discussed before, your natural waist is to be found at the smallest point of your torso. So from now on, never buy a dress with a fitted, seamed waist that doesn't hit you right at that exact spot. (You can thank me later!)

SHIFT: A shift dress is almost always sleeveless and cut to fall in a straight line down from the shoulders—not fitted to the body. Most shift dresses utilize small darts at the bust to add definition. This can result in an improper or too-tight fit across the chest if the darts hit the breasts at the incorrect spot.

STRAPLESS: A strapless dress is the trickiest style of dress to wear—but it has nothing to do with the size of your bust. The reason most strapless dresses won't stay up is lack of proper construction at the torso and waist, where the bulk of support is supposed to come from. If you have to tug on a strapless dress all night long, it's not providing proper support—which in plain English means (say it with me now!): *it doesn't fit!* You can help a strapless dress that doesn't have enough internal structure by wearing it with a longline bra (as discussed on page 139), but as you may know by now, a garment that doesn't fit you properly has no business taking up valuable real estate in your closet.

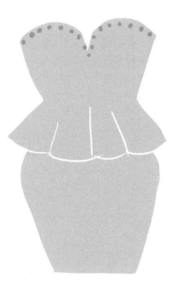

TANK: A tank-style dress is a good choice for those with narrower shoulders, as it is cut quite slim at the top. But beware of armholes that hang too low, exposing your bra to the world. Happily, a tank-style dress is an endlessly forgiving shape that is easy to have altered. A simple strap take-up (as discussed on page 34) can solve a too–low-slung tank dress in a jiffy.

WRAP: The wrap-style dress (made famous in the early 1970s by designer Diane von Furstenberg) is named for the front closure, which is formed by wrapping one side of the dress across the other and then tying them together at the side or back. They very much resemble the classic ballerina-style wrap top, but in dress form!

+ You've probably heard over and over that a wrap dress will fit every single woman perfectly due to its free-form nature. It's just too bad that couldn't be further from the truth! This is the biggest myth in fashion, because they almost never fit a smaller-busted woman properly. The deep plunge can easily slide between small breasts, causing the fabric to gape and sag. The small-breasted woman who wants to wear a wrap dress successfully will need to employ a safety pin, snap, or bit of Topstick (double-sided toupee tape, discussed on page 78) to keep the top half from falling open.

+ However, the classic wrap dress is a godsend for some larger-busted women, as it easily solves the problem of button-front style garments that won't close properly over large boobs. They are also a great choice for pregnant women, as the waist is bump-friendly and the bustline can accommodate wild fluctuations in bra size. But chances are, no matter what your body type, you're probably going to need a closure or a camisole to keep a wrap dress together up top.

Once you start paying close attention to fit and stop fooling yourself into buying things just because they happen to be "in style," you'll be amazed at how much better you look and feel in your clothes. A little bit of trend following is fine—and totally necessary to great style. But knowing what fits properly and only buying what works for you will always trump whatever is allegedly in fashion. The old idea that certain styles are definitively "in" or "out" is dated, tired, and just plain lame. Fashion is an industry that runs solely on dissatisfaction. We could easily take the whole thing down just by deciding to be happy with ourselves! And learning what works for you, fit-wise, and being happy with it is the key to real, lasting satisfaction with your style— clothing trends and glossy know-it-all fashion rags be damned.

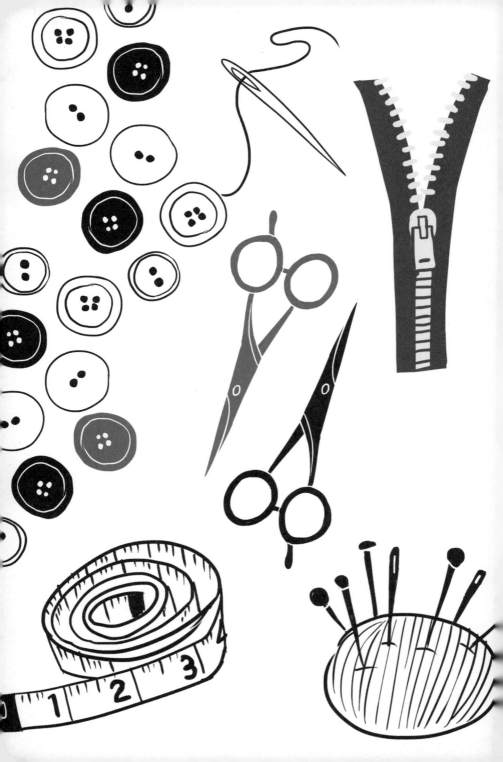

CHAPTER 3

ALTER YOUR CLOTHES,
alter your life

The most common complaint I hear from people about their clothes is that they don't ever fit them right. Pants are always too long, jackets too boxy, shirtsleeves way too voluminous, and dresses are forever just the tiniest bit too small. When I tell them to hush up and have their stuff tailored already, everyone acts like this is a shocking and foreign concept, available only to rich people or feudal lords—and pointless for the average human to even attempt. When clothes don't fit right off the rack, they just give up. It's a shame, because a nip here and a tuck there is sometimes all a garment needs to make the leap from an off-the-rack sad sack to an adorable, flattering work of art. A clever spot of tailoring can also reinvigorate clothes you already have but never wear due to simple, easily resolved fit issues.

What none of these people realize is that the idea of buying clothes in a store and expecting them to magically fit is actually quite new. A household's clothing was historically made by either professional tailors or family members until the mid-1920s, when the Industrial Revolution finally allowed the ready-made garment industry to explode. However, most of these new fangled "off-the-rack" garments that were suddenly sold in stores fit quite poorly, resulting in a steady stream of returns from unsatisfied customers and overall poor sales. This was due to the fact that early clothing manufacturers didn't have standardized sizes—in fact, they were almost arbitrary! Garments of wildly differing sizes were frequently labeled as being the same size by a multitude of manufacturers. (The more things change, the more they stay the same, right?)

It wasn't until the mid-1940s (after the U.S. Department of Agriculture finally conducted a study of body measurements) that a standard sizing system was created. But just as soon as this supposedly "standardized" sizing was put into place, vanity sizing came along in the 1950s and confused matters once again. (Of course, we couldn't even have five measly minutes until size became a hot-button, emotionally fraught issue.) Vanity sizing is why you always read that Marilyn

Monroe would wear a size twelve or fourteen by today's standards, when the clothes she wore in the 1950s were marked as size eight. The point of all this is that size tags in clothes have been more of a suggestion than an actual fact since day one—so it's not surprising that nothing ever fits anyone properly when they first try it on.

My great-great grandmother was a seamstress for the Ringling Bros. and Barnum & Bailey Circus in the early 1920s. Not only were her sewing skills legendary, her daughter, my great grandmother, learned how to sew under the big top, too—and as a result, she made the bulk of my clothes as a child (in addition to entire wardrobes for every doll I ever owned!) On the rare occasions my great grandmother did buy off-the-rack clothes for me in department stores, she still made simple alterations to them to ensure a perfect fit. To women of her generation, it was just something you did. But even when I was a wee child in the late 1980s, my great grandmother was already an incredibly ancient throwback to a far different era—because the 1970s had come along almost twenty years earlier and ushered in everything we now call modern life, including a whole new style of lackadaisical, ultracasual dressing. The freewheeling, flowing fashions of the groovy 1970s are what finally (and sadly) swept the idea of always tailoring one's clothes to fit properly right out the door—seemingly forever.

Take a minute to think about your favorite article of clothing. Why do you love it so much? Most likely, it's because it fits you as if it were made for you. Having a tailor you know and trust is still quite

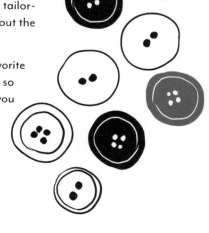

common in Europe, but for some reason, it's considered a luxury in the states. I believe you should actually plan to include tailoring in your wardrobe budget—if you want to look fantastic in your clothes, that is. Why do you think stars look like stars in their clothes? It's because there's a tailor and costume designer behind the scenes, altering absolutely every single garment they ever wear, right down to their T-shirts and camisoles. I've personally never, ever put an actor on camera in any piece of clothing that didn't have at least one alteration done to it. I realize this sounds crazy and un-achievable by mere mortals—but it's really not. Even though I alter every single thing my actors wear, it's usually something quite small—an alteration that would cost you less than twenty bucks at your local dry cleaner or tailor shop. And here's my real secret: I'm pretty much doing the same really easy alterations (or some variation thereof) over and over and over. Once you learn what they are and how to make them work for you, you'll become a pro at seeing just how easily certain garments can be finessed to fit your body perfectly.

THE TOTALLY WORTH-IT ALTERATIONS
YOU REALLY NEED TO KNOW ABOUT

Knowing how to spot an easy alteration is life changing. It opens up an entirely new world of clothes you previously thought you couldn't wear. Plus, you can likely salvage many of the ill-fitting garments you already own just by having them altered slightly—because really, any old garment will look miles better when it actually fits properly! But alterations aren't magic, nor will they transform every single poorly made, misshapen lump of a dress into a princess gown. And to justify the added cost of alterations, you'd better be in love with the garment in the first place. If you're on the fence, you shouldn't buy it—the cost of making alterations can easily exceed what you paid for it. Luckily, the alterations I'm about to share with you all happen to have a pretty low degree of difficulty—so you should be able to ask any tailor for them without fear—and for less than the cost of a nice dinner out.

SHORTEN A SHIRT OR ADD A SHIRTTAIL HEM

If every shirt you try on is so long that it could double as a dress, this is the alteration for you. Having a shirt hem taken up even a half inch can make a big difference; a too-long top can overwhelm a petite frame and always tends to bunch up and look sloppy. On most simple tops (even those with buttons), you can also ask your tailor to add a curved, shirttail-style hem instead of a boring straight one to create a more interesting, flattering silhouette. This alteration also allows you to tuck tops into clingier skirts or pants with only minimal bunching since there's less fabric to tuck in.

However, if there are pockets or zippers involved near the hem of the shirt, I'm sorry to say that attempting to shorten it probably isn't worth the trouble. Leave those pieces on the rack and never look back, because replacing zippers and moving pockets can become costly alterations. However, if there is a small amount of simple trim (such as lace or fringe) near the hem and you truly love the shirt, it may actually be worth the extra money a tailor will charge you to remove and reattach it while performing the alteration.

TAKE IN A SHIRT AT THE SIDE SEAMS

The golden rule of alterations is that anywhere a straight seam exists on a garment is pretty much fair game for an alteration. So if you're considering the purchase of a blouse you love with a fit that's on the not-so-perfect boxy side, check to see if it has a straight seam on each side of the body. If it does, march right up to the register and pay for that bad boy, because taking a straight seam in at the sides is one of the easiest clothing fixes there is. If your boxy-cut shirt has sleeves, the alteration becomes slightly more complicated because the tailor will need to cut into the underarm area, too. But altering the sides through the underarm is still easily enough accomplished and totally worth doing. Just keep in mind that it means you'll have to make sure the shirt in question has enough room in the underarm to allow for a small chunk of fabric to be removed. If it's big on the sides but tight in the underarm, it's a no-go.

TAKE UP A SHOULDER SEAM (OR SHORTEN YOUR STRAPS)

This is the mother of all alterations for those of you with short torsos. If you find that many garments hang down a little too low in front and show the sides of your bra, it's likely due to the shoulder seam being too long. (And a good shoulder fit is important; it can actually improve the look and feel of the entire garment.) This alteration works best with a sleeveless or tank top–style blouse, as removing the sleeves and reattaching them is tricky, and many times, they won't hang right afterward.

Taking a sleeveless garment up at the shoulder seam is an easy, inexpensive fix—however, it does automatically raise the front and back necklines, too, making the neckline circumference smaller (and whatever amount you raise the shoulder seam will also take the armhole up by the same amount), so make sure you can afford the room before you take the plunge. And remember: This simple fix is not for shoulders that fit poorly overall—nor for shoulder seams that extend past where your natural shoulder ends. It's strictly for garments that hang too low at the chest. An overall poorly fitted shoulder is a very bad thing, and it's not likely to get better, no matter how much tailoring you employ.

HEM A PAIR OF PANTS, A SKIRT, OR EVEN A DRESS

I've been in countless department store dressing rooms and overheard shopper after shopper decide not to purchase a pair of pants simply because they were too long in the leg. I'm always stunned and am forever running onto the sales floor half dressed to preach the gospel of hemming. A simple hem on a pair of pants should run you about $12—but the difference it makes in your look is priceless. A dragging hem billowing around your ankle throws off the entire line of your pants, causing them to bunch and crumple unflatteringly all the way up to your pockets. Just a few inches off the bottom allows the pants to fall straight from your hips as the designer intended—resulting in a clean, sleek, line from waist to floor.

The length you choose to hem your pants is a totally personal choice, and changes as styles come in and out of fashion. But for a pair of women's pants meant to be worn in a professional setting, you can't go wrong with having your hem fall between your heel and midshoe, breaking at about the mid-arch of your instep. You want the pant leg to hang straight—not bunch up at the top of your foot. By contrast, the proper break (meaning where your pants fall on your shoes) on a pair of men's pants is a little longer. I prefer a full-break pant length for men, which means you'll need to ask the tailor to adjust the length to hit right at the top of the shoe sole in back.

But what about jeans? Everyone thinks shortening the hem is totally out of the question because it's so hard to replicate the original one due to stitching details. But it's really not—you just need to turn your tailor on to the "Hollywood Hem." To achieve it, put on your jeans and figure out where you want the new length to be. Use a pin to mark the spot. Then, cuff the legs up (so they are inside out) until the original hem is right above your existing pin. Use another pin to secure the cuff into place. Take your jeans to the tailor and have them sew right below the original hem, taking care not to sew through any part of the original hem itself. Once it's stitched down, your tailor will cut off the bottom fold of excess fabric, flip the original hem down and press it into place. Your jeans will now fit properly and look as if they came from the store that way!

A word of warning: Always make sure to wash and dry your jeans at least once or twice before hemming so they can get all the shrinkage out of their system. Then, and only then, will you know how much you can safely chop off. If you're pressed for time, you can always fake a temporary hem using a bit of Topstick toupee tape and a prayer—just follow the instructions outlined on page 78!

ADD SOME DARTS

Do you have a skirt or pair of pants that's just a little bit too big in the waist but fits nicely through the hips and thighs? This commonly occurs because a woman's body is generally wider at the hips than at the waist. It can be remedied by simply slapping two darts (small folds sewn into fabric that help provide shape to a garment) in at the back waistband, nipping the gap in the bud—and shaping the garment to fit you like a glove. Darts are most commonly used in blouses to improve fit at the bustline, but I find them to be just as useful to shape a pair of pants or a skirt. The tailor will space the two darts evenly apart, most likely placing them over the fullest part of each bum cheek. The darts will take in the most fabric at the waistband and go down to zero fabric at the point where your hips begin to widen. Darts aren't all that tricky, but they do take a bit of skill—so this alteration will likely run you about $20 to $25.

You can also use darts to slim down a boxy jacket. If you have broad shoulders, you may find that you need to buy your jackets a size or two up to have them fit well through the shoulders—but this almost always causes it to be too boxy through the waist. Ask your tailor to open up the jacket's lining and add two darts at the jacket's back, starting right behind the sleeves and ending just before the hem for about $40.

Some tailors will refuse to do this alteration on a highly structured jacket, as the "proper" way to slim a complicated jacket is from the side seams, which usually necessitates moving pockets—a far more costly alteration. But adding darts at the back of a simply constructed jacket is a quick fix that is well worth the money—because even though it's a relatively easy alteration, it tends to make it look like it was precision tailored to your body.

SLIM DOWN A SLEEVE

Cutting down a voluminous sleeve is another alteration that doesn't cost a ton but makes a huge difference in how a garment looks. When a sleeve is too loose, it usually means that the armpit is too big as well. Your tailor can take in anywhere from a half inch to a full two inches from the underside sleeve seam, going from the wrist all the way to the underarm and down into the side-boob seam to create a slimmed down, prettier shape.

Your tailor may try to tell you that he or she needs to actually remove the sleeves from the garment to "properly" take in the sleeve and underarm area, but the shortcut method outlined above is one I've used for years with great success—and sometimes all you really need is the fastest, least expensive way to get from point A to point B. Just make sure you can actually bend your arm at the elbow with the proposed sleeve alteration before the tailor stitches it up for good. I learned this lesson the hard way when I accidentally altered an actor's sleeves way too tight and only found out about it minutes before she was meant to be in a scene that called for her to wave her arms above her head in a dramatic fashion. Actors are troopers though—when the director called *"Action!"* she hunched her shoulders up and waved her arms around like a champ—without anybody ever noticing that she wasn't actually able to bend them at all.

TAPER A TROUSER LEG

You obviously can't make a pair of wide-leg pants into a legging with this alteration, but you can have your tailor easily trim a bit of excess volume along the garment's inner and outer seams, resulting in a more streamlined silhouette. However, fair warning: Bringing a pair of pants in by more than about two inches often necessitates moving the pockets to a point where the whole thing just looks wrong. While it is technically possible to take in a pair of pants that are many sizes too big, it's far beyond the realm of what I'd call a "simple" alteration—and a tailor will charge you accordingly. You may be better off just springing for a new pair that fits you better.

REPLACE A TERRIBLE INVISIBLE ZIPPER

The zipper is an amazing mechanical invention that makes fastening one's clothes easier than our nineteenth-century counterparts could ever have imagined. Before the modern zipper burst onto the scene around 1920, clothes-wearers the world over were stuck fumbling with buttons and tediously fastening hook and eye closures. But as with all mechanical inventions, zippers sometimes break or don't always work exactly as they should. The zipper that will give you the most trouble in life is an invisible zipper, which is practically embedded into the garment, rendering the zipper—wait for it—invisible once zipped up! They are commonly found on better cocktail and party dresses, and practically every garment I've ever bought that has one tends to get stuck right over the rib cage or manage to munch all the fabric in its path, rendering the item completely unusable.

Actors always have a moment of panic when a garment with an invisible zipper won't close, thinking it means the dress is too small—but what it really means is that the zipper is either of poor quality or has been installed improperly. The dollar amount you pay for a garment doesn't spare you from a crummy zipper, either. I've seen it happen with garments that cost less than twenty bucks all the way up to a $4,000 wedding gown. Most of the time, this problem occurs because the zipper has been sewn too close to the fabric edge. This problem is *especially* deadly when it occurs at a pressure point, like over the boobs or at the ribcage. The end result is always the same—pinched skin and a broken zipper.

I spend the twenty to thirty bucks it costs and take every single inexpensive invisible-zippered garment I buy to the tailor and ask that it be replaced with a zipper of better quality (as the zipper on a $20.00 dress likely cost $0.50—and is therefore incredibly prone to breaking), paying close attention to the spots where zippers are known to get stuck. But sometimes, the existing zipper can actually just be eased out a bit along the points where it is sticking by having your tailor scoot the tape (the fabric on either side of the teeth) over just a few centimeters, thereby getting the teeth out of the way of the fabric and ensuring a smooth zip. A zipper alteration is totally worth the money—every single time.

If you are asking your tailor to replace the zipper completely, you may need to provide them with the new zipper to ensure a perfect color and style match. This means a trip to the fabric store is in your future—and once you are there, spring for the very best zipper money can buy. I like to replace all plastic zippers with metal ones; they are stronger and can take more of a beating. Oh—and be sure to bring the garment to the store with you so you aren't left scratching your head, wondering which zipper is a better match. The rule of color matching a zipper to a dress is this: Close is always good enough. Once you're zipped up, the zipper becomes practically invisible. So nobody's going to know if your dress is dusty orange—but your zipper happens to be a little closer to pale peach. A replacement zipper is in the neighborhood of $8 to purchase, and a tailor will charge you about $12 to install it.

If you have a dress that's just a few centimeters too tight (or every zipper you ever use breaks and gets stuck), you could also consider replacing your invisible zippers with a sturdier exposed zipper and treating it like a style detail. An easy-to-use exposed zipper means you'll never find yourself rushing into a party with your dress unzipped, looking for two people to help you—one to zip and one to hold the sides together. (For more tips on zipper maintenance, plus what to do when one eventually breaks on you, turn to page 85.)

BUT SOMETIMES, IT'S JUST NOT WORTH IT

Now the bad news: There are certain alterations that I don't believe are ever worth pursuing, due to a poor return on your time and money investment. The truth is that some garments are just badly designed—and no amount of tailoring, no matter how skilled, can make up for that.

A VERY BAD ARMHOLE

The point where the sleeve meets the armhole is called the "armscye" and is the most important part of any garment. A poorly set armhole can ruin an entire frock in an instant—and is almost impossible to fix. Have a good, long, hard look at how a garment fits at the armhole while in the store before you drop your hard-earned money on it, because that will be the thing that stops you from wearing it every time you reach for it in your closet. Paying a tailor to attempt a fix on a badly set armhole is the very definition of throwing good money after bad.

A TOO-LONG JACKET SLEEVE OR BODY

A suit jacket or blazer that is too long in the body or arms can be a money pit to have altered. Shortening a sleeve entails removing the buttons at the wrist in addition to the lining inside the jacket. Also, most suit jackets have a small vent at each cuff, further complicating a sleeve alteration. While it's not terribly difficult, it is time consuming, which equals a higher cost—so I don't recommend doing it unless the jacket is something that you really, really love. A jacket that is too long in the body is an equally deadly alteration because the distance from the top of the pockets to the bottom of the jacket is a rather exact science. Shortening a jacket's hem more than about an inch throws the entire look of the garment off. Remember back when I said that a straight seam is fair game for an easy alteration? Well, a curved jacket hem is the exact opposite of a straight seam, and you can be sure that any tailor will charge you accordingly.

A TOO-SMALL GARMENT

If you are even considering whether or not a tailor can let out a garment that is just a hair too small, you need to answer one question before anything else: Does the item in question have enough fabric to do so? You can determine this by having a peek at the inside seams in the area where the garment is too snug. If there is at least one-half to one inch of extra fabric lurking on either side of the seams, you can sometimes have the garment let out by just about that amount. But even the best tailor in the world can't help you if the fabric isn't there. Larger seam allowances are standard on newer clothing, but vintage items can sometimes have far less. I am of the opinion that if it's more than just a smidge too tight, forget it—because it is highly unlikely that it can be easily and cheaply expanded.

ANYTHING PLEATED, SEQUINED, BEADED, OR MADE OF LACE OR CHIFFON

Very intricate pieces with heavy beading or sequins will cost more to alter, as the fabric requires more care and time to sew. A tailor almost always has to do these alterations by hand, because beads and sequins get stuck in a sewing machine quite easily—and the minute you cut into anything with embellishments, you are likely to see those beads and sequins start unraveling themselves and rolling onto the floor.

Chiffon pieces also require a higher degree of concentration and skill to alter properly—the delicate nature of the fabric makes errant needle holes very obvious, so it has to be done perfectly the first time. Lace is in the same difficulty category as chiffon; the open weave can get sucked into a sewing machine quite easily. For this reason, most tailors sew lace and chiffon by hand—and you guessed it, that's going to cost you more money. Garments that are pleated or have a scalloped edge also require more skill to tailor—and will be priced accordingly.

ANYTHING WITH A LINING

A garment with lining means your tailor is doing double the work, because the lining is really like a second garment! Lining can also sometimes misbehave and become twisted once altered, so consider how much you really love something before buying it if it's constructed with lining and needs an alteration. The exception to this rule is getting rips in lining replaced—which is an easy fix and well worth the time and effort.

A LEATHER OR SUEDE GARMENT

Tailors have to use special needles (and sometimes special machines as well) to alter leather and suede pieces. Also, leather isn't the same as fabric—it's a hide, so it has weak points here and there that sometimes don't become obvious until you cut into them. You can't make a mistake when sewing a hide—as the needle holes can't be hidden. I don't attempt to alter leather pieces much further than a simple hem here and there, as it ends up being rather costly. Altering a leather piece you already own is another story and can sometimes create a beautiful garment from one that was just gathering dust—but buying an expensive leather item brand new and then spending even more money to have it tailored is a rich person's game. Play it at your own peril.

HOW TO FIND A GREAT TAILOR

There's one giant catch to all of this: Not one word of what I just told you matters if you don't have a good tailor on speed dial. Lots of folks call themselves tailors, but that doesn't mean they are skilled. Finding a tailor you trust is just like any other relationship—sometimes you have to kiss a lot of frogs until you find "the one." But finding the one isn't all that hard once you know how to go about it:

42

+ Pick someone who is nice. Some tailors can be cantankerous and downright mean—but the fact that you are asking them to perform a service you kind of know nothing about doesn't give them an excuse to be snappy. Skip any tailor who gives you attitude in your initial meeting—because you are looking to form a relationship with someone who has your wardrobe's best interests at heart. No amount of magical sewing can make up for mean, bad service.

+ Seek recommendations. I had to ask at least twenty people for recommendations before I found my current alterations wizard. (And I'm a professional clothes-handler!) Friends and family are a good place to start, but don't hesitate to ask salesclerks, dry cleaners, and boutique employees who they like and recommend.

+ Look for a tailor who takes appointments. This means they take their job seriously and will take the time to answer your questions. Walk-in spots can be good in a pinch, but you're really looking to build a working relationship.

+ Search out a tailor who understands style. Your tailor needn't be a runway model in Paris, but a working knowledge of current trends and style cues is invaluable in bridging the gap between what you want and what is physically possible. A good tailor should point out when what you are asking for defies the laws of physics or classic style. Whether or not you decide to press on with an alteration after a tailor suggests you don't is entirely up to you. I've had a few happy accidents this way, but more often than not, my tailor was right when he or she told me that what I wanted was just plain crazy.

+ Make sure the tailor is available. You want a tailor who is accessible when you find out the day before a wedding that your once well-fitting dress or suit needs a bit of emergency help. While good tailors are often booked far in advance, you want someone who can make time to help you out of a jam.

+ Examine their handiwork. Once you get your first piece back from a tailor, look not only at the outside of the garment, but also at the inside stitching and overall work. Make sure everything lines up, that seams are even, and that thread ends are knotted securely so as to prevent premature unraveling. Having an inexpensive simple hem done is a good test before you send something more complicated to a new tailor.

+ Educate yourself. Know what you want, and don't be afraid to ask questions. Learn the terms for basic alterations (listed below) so you can better communicate with your tailor.

So, what about those people who say they can buy clothes right off the rack and have them fit perfectly, as if they were made just for them? They are as rare as magical unicorns—which means they don't actually exist.

BASIC TAILORING TERMS

TAKE IN: If a dress, skirt, or pair of pants is too wide in the waist-line, you can ask a tailor to take it in. A loose-fitting blouse bodice or sleeve can also be taken in at the side seams. But if a garment is taken in more than about three or four inches, you may be left with unbalanced results.

LET OUT: Sometimes all you need is an extra half inch or so in the waistline or at the hem of a pair of pants or dress to render the garment perfect. However, there needs to be enough fabric in the garment to be let out in the first place—so when considering having an item let out, have a close look at the seams, keeping in mind that you'll need to leave at least a half inch on either side of each seam for stability's sake. You can't sew a fabric edge right up to the seam if you have any plans to walk, dance, move, or breathe in the garment! Letting out is a bit trickier than taking in.

BRING UP: The too-long sleeves of a blouse can easily be brought up by about three inches—as long as any buttons at the wrist will not interfere. Pant hems can also be brought up about three inches—just be sure it does not then cause the pants to lose their shape. Sleeves and pant hems can almost never be "brought-down," so stay far away from items that are too short.

REPAIR: This is a blanket term you can use with a tailor anytime you want a particular mechanical piece of a garment restored to its former glory: "zipper repair," "button repair," "belt loop repair," and so on.

MEND A SEAM: When seams start to tear apart on a dress, pair of pants, or lining of a jacket, you can ask your tailor to mend the seam for you. Mending will close the gap and incorporate the repair into the original seam stitching.

ADD DARTS: Darts are folds sewn into fabric with the intent to enhance the wearer's shape. Darts are most commonly found in women's blouses and dresses at the bust line to help give shape to the figure.

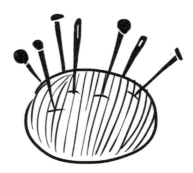

DARN: Holes in knit sweaters, shirts, or scarves can be repaired by a tailor who specializes in darning, which is the art of re-weaving small, matching bits of yarn into the hole. Darning is quickly becoming a lost art, so you may have to search far and wide for a tailor who specializes in mending knitted items.

TAPER: The term "tapering" is usually used to describe the narrowing of a pant leg. To successfully taper a pair of pants, the alteration must run from hip to hem—not just from below the knee down. Otherwise, you'll wind up with slacks that look like genie trousers.

Don't fool yourself into thinking that having something altered is a once-in-a-lifetime deal, meant only for wedding gowns and other fancy occasion wear. A nip here and a tuck there (also known as a facelift for your wardrobe!) could be all that's standing between a good outfit and a great one—so what are you waiting for?

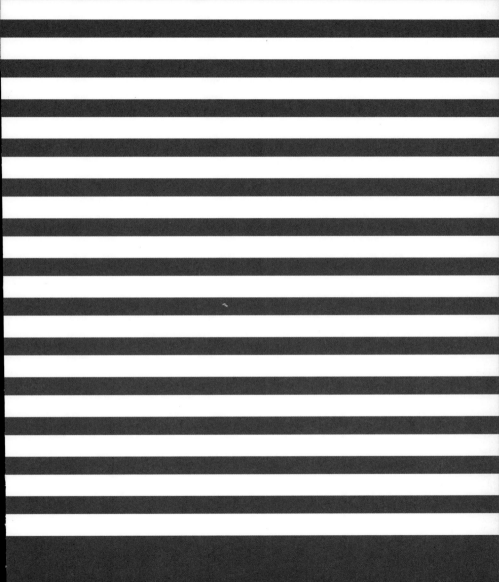

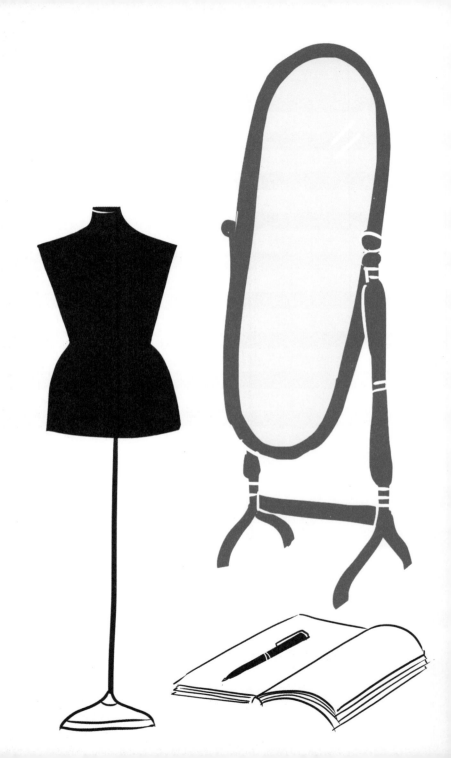

CHAPTER
4

BE YOUR OWN
costume designer

You already know that good clothes really do open all doors. That's not to say that your clothes need to be fancy, expensive, or even any particular style. But they are the first thing people judge you on, and your clothes say a lot about you before you even open your mouth. So it's important to be the boss lady in charge of what your style is saying about you behind your back. This means you should spend at least a little time acting as your own costume designer, figuring out your "signature style." I know a handful of people who have their signature styles down cold—I could take one glance at one of them from the back on a crowded street and instantly know, "Oh yeah, that's her." But how did they get their styles? The answer is that they most likely gave it to themselves. Taking the time to figure out your own signature style is something most people have never considered doing, but it's a great tool to have at your disposal if you often find yourself in a dressing room, uncertain if something works for you, reduced to texting photos of a dress to all your pals with the question: "Should I buy this? Yes or no?" Because that's all style really is—a tool. When used wisely, it removes doubt from getting dressed and can make you feel cooler, smarter, sexier, and stronger. Who doesn't want that?

YOUR STYLE IS YOUR SIGNATURE

Finding your signature style only sounds like something that takes a lifetime to accomplish. It's actually pretty easy and lots of fun! The end goal is to come up with a few words or a clever, visual phrase that really sums up who you are as a person. You can then lean on that phrase while shopping or getting dressed each morning. It becomes a lens to filter how the world views you—and more importantly, how you view yourself. But why do you need to bother finding your signature style, anyway? It's obviously not vital to our continued survival, but there is inherent value and power in knowing what you are projecting to the world every time you get dressed. That's the main reason I have a job dressing people who are in the public eye—clothes are instant visual cues to who a person is, where they came from, and where they may be going.

To get started, make a list of all the things you like. This list can include absolutely anything that moves you, because there's way more to having a signature style than just the clothes you wear. I believe it's actually a combination of the history, art, music, food, hobbies, and culture that speak to you. In the beginning stages of sleuthing out what your signature style really is, write down everything you can think of that interests you as a jumping off point to delve into what your core style may be. This is my exact process to figure out a character's look on a show, by the way—I break out an old-fashioned yellow legal pad and force myself to think like the character. What books does she like? What things does she hold sacred? What's her favorite color? What types of art does she gravitate toward? I write it all down, and a clear picture of the character starts to appear, slowly but surely. When you apply this process to yourself, you're actually acting as your own costume designer! And you might be surprised where your character's style exploration leads you.

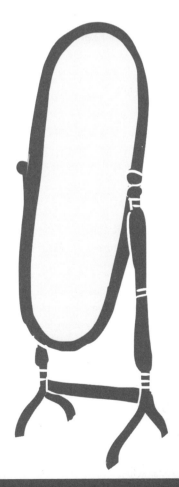

Here's my personal style study as an example: I am a proud Texan. (There is no other kind of Texan, actually!) There isn't a day that goes by that I don't miss and think fondly of my home state. So cowboy boots and country-girl style are always going to work their way into my look. But I'm also a die-hard new-waver—the very first concert I ever saw was Depeche Mode. My entire high school career was spent wearing black knee-high socks, black suspenders, and my grandfather's old black trousers that I chopped at the knee to show off my socks. I also sported a pretty sweet bi-level, asymmetrical "wedge" haircut in a town where cheerleaders with ribbons in their ponytails were the ideal of beauty. As a result, black and edgy pieces will always find their way into my closet, no matter what I try to do. It's practically genetic at this point. But my love for country-tinged looks is never-ending as well, so I call my current style "Backwoods Nouveau." It means that my go-to slouching around town look is usually a pair of leather-trimmed jeans, a snap-front western inspired shirt, and brightly colored ankle boots with simple, poppy details. Sometimes I swap in cowboy boots and an old T-shirt—making sure to pile on some colorful, geometric plastic jewelry to give the cowboy boots that missing new-wave edge.

Whatever your signature style, it can definitely change and grow—you can even have two at once! Whenever I'm feeling the need to "grow up" my professional look a bit, I find myself inexplicably drawn to very classic, heavily tailored pieces. I've also started properly reading the books I only skimmed in high school—*Anna Karenina*, *Jane Eyre,* and *Madame Bovary*. I've even found myself suddenly wanting to listen to classical music in my office while I work! Which is all terrifying, as I've always prided myself on being edgy and against the grain. But I've decided to give in to my ladylike-loving side a bit—just being sure to always temper it with something slightly bizarre. As a result, I'm calling my secondary signature style "Genteel Bizarro." (I got that from consulting my trusty thesaurus for synonyms for both "ladylike" and "weird.")

What does it mean style-wise? It means that I've started buying simple sheath dresses and tempering their classic, conservative edge with downright creepy jewelry like gold eyeball earrings and knife rings. The resulting mash up is a look that doesn't hit you over the head at first glance, but reveals itself over the course of a conversation. It's great to go to a business meeting and watch people notice the subtle yet slightly gory details of my otherwise perfect ladylike outfits.

Figuring out your own signature style isn't as hard as it may seem. Practically any keywords that you identify with can be melded into a signature style—because there's actually way more to having a signature style than just the clothes you wear. You can use almost anything that interests you as a jumping off point to delve into what your core style may be. This exercise is an excellent way to get your wheels turning as to what really floats your style boat. Get a pen, paper, and your thesaurus (I swear, it helps!) and spend some time laser-focusing your current or aspirational signature style down to just two or three words. You want to get to the heart of who you are, what interests you, and what you really want to present to the world before you allow yourself to go forth and shop. Your signature style can be as simple or fantastical as you want it to be.

Here are some real-life examples from some of my online readers who took on this challenge:

LIBRARIAN NOIR, EMILY, TWENTY-FIVE YEARS OLD: "I run the library at my local university, so proper bookish styles have always been the cornerstone of my personal style. But the older I get, the more I find myself wanting to break out of the classic 'librarian' mold. I still need to look professional—I'm just looking to add a bit of zip to my existing work clothes. After writing down all the books and films I love, I realized that what I really wanted was to add a little classic Hollywood sex appeal to my wardrobe. That's how I ended up with 'Librarian Noir.' I've plugged a few fluffy angora sweaters and seamed stockings into my existing closet of pencil skirts and ballet flats. The result is a look that signals to the world that I'm a very proper lady—with a few secrets hidden just beneath the surface, should one want to scratch."

CLASSIC POP, SHARON, THIRTY-FIVE YEARS OLD: "I've read thousands of words on why every woman should own a little black dress, the perfect white shirt, or a classic trench coat to always be well dressed. The older I get, the more I want to be taken 'seriously,' but those classics always seem too boring and staid—so not 'me.' I am drawn toward garments with clean, unfussy lines but love colors that pop above all else. After writing down all the disparate things I like, I realized that what I should be shopping for are classic garments in those crazy, poppy colors that I naturally gravitate toward—like a hot pink trench coat or a cashmere sweater in bright chartreuse green. These colorful, simple basics satisfy my need for color and provide a backdrop for the other parts of my outfit to really sing."

FAUX BESPOKE, DAISY, TWENTY-NINE YEARS OLD: "I used an online thesaurus (it totally helps!) to find synonyms for 'custom-made' and ended up with 'bespoke.' I like my stuff to look like it has been made just for me—even though I can't afford one-of-a-kind things, hence the 'faux!' I've started collecting photos of high-end, custom-made pieces and studying their fabrication. As a result, I can now immediately eagle-eye a garment with unique, unusual details in a sea of look-alike pieces. The things I've bought since defining my style have all been under $35, but my coworkers have started asking me if I've learned to sew due to my new, "unique" wardrobe. I don't have the heart to tell them the truth!"

AUSTERE GLAM, JACKIE, FIFTY YEARS OLD: "Growing up in Sweden, I was exposed to lots of sleek, sharp, severe clothing design. It's what I've always worn, and it matches my no-nonsense personality perfectly. But upon moving to the States, I developed a serious obsession with 1970s glitter rock and all the glam it entails. I never seriously thought about the fact that I could express this in my personal style until I wrote it down on my list of things I love—and as a result, I've started working some luxe, metallic accessories into my everyday look. In the middle of a stressful day, those bright and shiny pieces remind me of who I am—and that there's more to life than whatever troubles I'm dealing with at the moment."

Now that you have an idea of how some readers have defined, refined, and named their signature styles, you can get down to the business of figuring out your own. Once you've got yours, start using it as a filter to determine if the item you are looking to purchase really suits you or not. It may seem slightly ridiculous, but putting together a journal or collage of images that illustrate the idea of your new signature style phrase will also help your brain wrap itself around what to keep your eyes peeled for when you are out shopping. Collecting images may also lead you to consider styles you wouldn't previously have thought of, which is what usually happens to me. I tear pages out of magazines, bookmark things I could never afford on fancy retail websites, and snap photos of stuff in stores while I am out shopping for work. When I glance at this catalog of images, a pattern usually starts to emerge, and I can see more clearly what styles I am really drawn to. It's a way of editing down what you like and what works for you before you make the commitment to buy something— much like researching the pros and cons of a new car purchase in advance of actually bringing it home. Approaching your wardrobe like the investment it is can help cut down on the number of unworn, unloved items hanging in your closet.

HOW TO SEARCH OUT PIECES
THAT ARE SO TOTALLY YOU

Keeping an eye on high-end styles and looks from places that aren't in your budget may sound like torture—but it's actually an excellent way to know what to keep looking for when shopping elsewhere. Copycat fashion stores are here to stay, and being able to spot wallet-friendly pieces that are inspired by more expensive versions is one of the main secrets to being superstylish on a shoestring budget. When you keep track of what the big designers are doing, it becomes easy to snap up things that are in your style wheelhouse wherever you find them—at a thrift store, a clearance rack at the mall, or your local dollar store. (Don't laugh— I do indeed have pieces in my closet that I snagged for a buck while looking for deals on household goods.) That's the ultimate secret to having good personal style: Once you've established what you are looking for, be on the lookout for it everywhere, even in the most unlikely places (including the grocery store, your friends' closets, or on your coworkers' backs!). Recognizing good design wherever you happen to spot it is definitely a skill that can be learned—you just have to be willing to do the legwork.

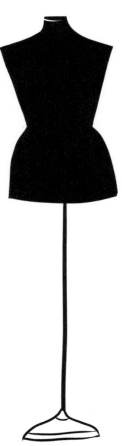

Also, don't be afraid to ask women on the street whose style you admire where they got something. Everyone likes to be compli- mented, and I find that a casual, "You look so great in what you're wearing!" followed by, "Would you be so kind as to tell me where you got it?" almost always results in them giving up the goods. Just be sure to have a stock response ready for the fancy babes who answer, "At Barney's," or "Oh, on vacation in Paris," so as not to feel like an instant hick. I always reply with a simple, "Nicely done!" (And then tuck the image of whatever they are wearing away in my mental file in case I see a great knockoff of it elsewhere at a price I can afford.) Having a signature style means that you are constantly on the lookout for what's new, fresh, and cool that actually suits you—so you can work it into your closet and not feel like you're trying on a personality. When you are your own costume designer, you'll find you are suddenly the very best version of yourself you've ever been. Because real style is all about enhancing who you already are—not attempting to change yourself into someone else.

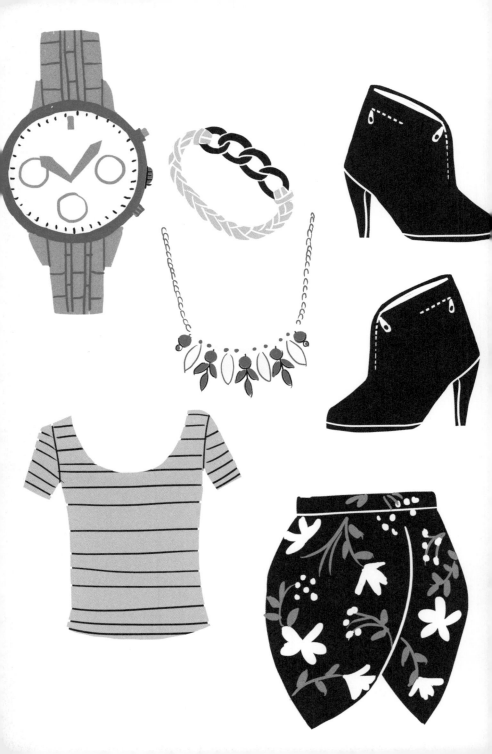

CHAPTER
5

DUMB
FASHION
RULES
*that were made
for breaking*

As a natural-born scofflaw, I despise almost all rules. And rules in fashion are particularly infuriating. Most of them are meant to trick us into dressing and acting exactly alike, which is dumb. I've always thought the "don'ts" in the back of magazines looked far more interesting than the perfect models on the preceding pages. The idea that "women should refrain from wearing shorter skirts past age forty," or that we should all "avoid wearing red with pink" is, in a word, totally boring. (Yeah, that's two words, but forget the rules, remember?)

Having great style is all about being different, unique, and, above all else, interesting. (Plus, wearing whatever the hell you want every day is at least five hundred times easier than remembering a bunch of antiquated dos and don'ts.) But if you need some extra reassuring, here are my top ten really dumb fashion rules that you should definitely toss into the wind without a care—because really, who's going to stop you?

DUMB RULE NUMBER ONE: ALWAYS FEAR WEARING STRIPES— HORIZONTAL OR OTHERWISE

I've had hundreds, if not thousands, of heated conversations with actors who are stuck believing this outdated rule. The old wisdom has always been that vertical stripes are more flattering than horizontal ones, but you might be surprised to find that the exact opposite is true. When your eye looks at vertical stripes on a body, it has to do a lot of work to take in the breadth of contrast. That's because when viewed from head to toe, vertical stripes warp where they skim over the wearer's breasts, hips, and shoulders, causing the brain to work harder to process what it is seeing. All this extra thinking then fools the brain into believing that the area is bigger than it actually is. But when the stripes run from left to right, there's a single unbroken line— so there's zero shape confusion for the brain to sort out. Because when the brain glosses over a detail, the eye does, too!

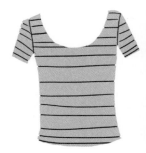

What *is* true is that the skinnier the stripe, the more the eye is fooled. A good equation to follow for stripe placement is 10 percent of the darker color and 90 percent of the lighter. But in the end, it's really the fit of the garment, not the width or placement of the stripes that determines if it works for you or not. And that is something only you can answer—no antiquated rules can help you figure it out. The bottom line is this: if you like stripes, then wear them without fear!

DUMB RULE NUMBER TWO: DON'T WEAR WHITE AFTER LABOR DAY

This rule was originally "Don't wear white shoes after Labor Day" but has somehow expanded to include white clothing as well. There are many theories as to how it actually became a rule—some say it was a way to show that one was a member of the leisure class and could afford to have an entire, separate summer-specific wardrobe. Fashion magazines of the early 1900s really cemented this rule in their editorial pages, likely in an attempt to keep Madame So-and-So from sullying her pristine summer lawn-party ensembles with mud from the heavy fall rains.

The laughable part of this made-up "rule" is that the real tastemakers of the day didn't subscribe to this theory even back then. Coco Chanel herself wore white year-round! And how else do you explain "winter whites"? I'd suggest avoiding linen, seersucker, and other very summer-specific fabrics in the winter, but other than that, it's game on for white clothes whenever you feel like looking angelic. (And if white is only acceptable for a few months out of the year, then why is a crisp white blouse on every single "must-have wardrobe items" list written since time immemorial?)

As for the white shoes, they *are* a bit of a challenge to keep clean in inclement weather. But the sense of lightness they give a dull winter outfit is well worth the hassle. As long as they aren't open-toed and strappy, I say you should slog through the slush in the middle of January in your white shoes and be happy—because it's really nobody's business what you do to please yourself.

DUMB RULE NUMBER THREE:
DON'T WEAR BLACK WITH BROWN OR NAVY

Hear me now: A brown belt is always the perfect foil for a black dress. It adds a sense of lightness that a solid black dress is inherently missing—while keeping the overall look low-key. Just make sure it's a lighter shade of brown for maximum contrast and always repeat a spot of brown somewhere else in your outfit, whether it's a leather cuff, a cardigan, your shoes, or your handbag.

And exactly what color shoe are you supposed to wear with a navy dress—matchy-matchy navy ones? Black footwear works well with navy or blue-black garments, but the real truth is that a black shoe grounds almost any outfit and gives it the sharp edge that a dainty, matching shoe never can. You can also successfully pair a cognac, tan, or oxblood shoe with any navy frock for a very chic Italian street–style look. Try it—I bet you'll like it!

DUMB RULE NUMBER FOUR:
DON'T MIX YOUR METALS

Mixing jewelry metals is not only okay, it's awesome. The more the merrier! A brilliant melody of metal tones is the total cool-girl secret to laid-back, laissez-faire style. If it wasn't, then how do you explain the enduring popularity of the Cartier "Trinity" ring, a classic since 1924 that consists of interlocking bands of pink, yellow, and white gold? But there's a secret to pulling it off—and it lies in always wearing a third piece that matches one you already have on, so it's not just a silver ring with a pair of gold earrings. You need to then add either a handbag with gold hardware or a necklace in silver to even out the look. I find that a simple set of bangles that mix silver and gold together give you an instant license to wear any other mixed metal colors you want at the same time.

Also, try adding a pinch of rose gold to your current jewelry rotation. It has a warm, luscious quality that goes with everything and flatters all skin tones. Look for a rose gold–hued ring or pair of stud earrings you can wear every day and plug other metals in with it at will. It's a great way to ease yourself into being a metal mixer!

DUMB RULE NUMBER FIVE: DON'T WEAR LEGGINGS AS PANTS

Here's the fashion world's most boring question: "Are leggings pants?" Of course they are! You can't keep people from loving a single gar-ment that can take you from your bed, to the gym, to work, then out to dinner, and back to bed with ease. Sure, we've all been exposed to a certain amount of shocking information about other people's private regions due to some too-sheer, too-tight pairs of leggings, but it's a small price to pay for such supreme comfort. I personally strive to pair my leggings with tops that at least graze my pubic bone, but it's really your divine right to wear yours as you see fit.

If you are a staunch defender of the "leggings aren't pants" rule, do yourself a favor and look into trying a double-knit pair, commonly known as ponte pants. They are a bit thicker and firmer than regular leggings but are just as comfy and stretchy. Ponte pants often have pockets or zippers, further legitimizing their status as actual pants—that just so happen to be crazy comfortable!

Before you leave the house, check your leggings for sheerness by taking a test photo of your backside using your phone's camera. Be sure to turn on the flash—because the harsh light of day reveals secrets that your dimly lit bedroom wants to keep from you. If there is any hint of sheerness, layer a long, bum-covering tank under your shirt to keep your assets under wraps. (And don't forget to delete those photos ASAP!) The making of leggings that are too sheer at the backside should be considered a crime—punishable by many years of hard labor, all overseen by the affected women.

DUMB RULE NUMBER SIX:
DON'T WEAR BOOTS IN THE SUMMER

The person who decreed this to be a fashion "rule" has obviously never had the misfortune of rolling an entire wardrobe rack full of clothes over the top of his or her bare flip-flopped foot. Life is inherently dangerous, and a great pair of boots helps protect your tootsies from harm. I wear boots to work every single day (no matter what the weather) after breaking half my toes in the aforementioned rack mishap. The trick is to make them look warm weather–appropriate and not cause passersby to wonder how much your feet must be sweating. (Although really, they should just mind their own darn business.) Keeping your boots at ankle height, your legs totally bare, and avoiding socks that look heavy or knitted usually does the trick. Choosing a pair of boots in a pale color to drive home the summertime vibe also keeps the overall look from becoming too wintry. Taller boots can work in the summertime, too—but always with taller socks or even sheer knee-highs to avoid gruesome shin sweat!

DUMB RULE NUMBER SEVEN: SHORT BOOTS
MAKE YOUR LEGS LOOK STUMPY

If you have sturdier legs, it's true that a pair of boots that hits you at midcalf is not the best choice. (They can also tend to overwhelm a petite frame.) But boots that hit right at the anklebone flatter every single body type there ever was. If you're concerned about drawing too much attention to your legs, look for a simple boot without a ton of embellishment—and pair them with knee socks to ape the look of taller boots if you need to ease yourself into feeling comfortable going bare-legged with them. I also think ankle boots on shorter legs can actually fool the eye into thinking the reason your legs look shorter is due to the boots—and not the other way around.

DUMB RULE NUMBER EIGHT:
DON'T MIX YOUR PATTERNS

Wearing contrasting patterns used to be dismissively called "clashing" and was something we were all advised to avoid. But truly fashionable women know that the secret to incredible style lies in knowing how to effortlessly mix patterns without going overboard. It's also a great way to expand your closet without spending a dime. If the secrets of masterful pattern mixing seem impossible to crack, I'm not surprised—when it goes wrong, it goes really, horribly wrong. Luckily there are some simple guidelines you can follow to achieve the perfect "mismatched" look—and they are almost impossible to mess up:

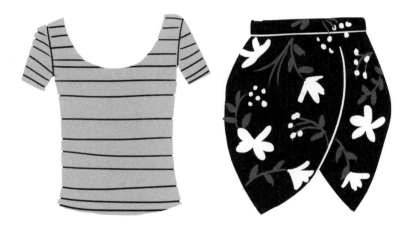

+ Keep it in the same color family. A head-to-toe solid-color outfit can veer into Jolly Green Giant territory very quickly—but a monochromatic color story is actually a great way to test the pattern-mixing waters while still maintaining a cohesive look. It's also a safe way to try your hand at pattern mixing in a conservative workplace. If you're a beginner, choose neutral-colored pieces (like brown or

HOW TO GET DRESSED

nude) done up in perky florals and zesty zigzags. Play it safe with
your shoes, both in style and color, until you get your sea legs.

+ Echo the color of one pattern in the other. If you're wearing a
floral patterned shirt with a navy background on your top half,
choose a skirt that incorporates a navy stripe for the bottom.
The repeating color helps tone down the overall look and adds
a sense of cohesiveness that can feel missing from some mixed-
pattern masterpieces. (It's also a good trick to fall back on
when all else fails!)

+ Treat houndstooth, polka dots, thin stripes, and checks as solids.
Classic, repeating patterns work beautifully when they are
small and understated enough that your eye can understand
them as solid colors—even though they obviously are not! This
includes highly textured fabrics like nubby, Chanel-esque tweed
pieces. Wear your favorite ultraclassic patterns as if they are
solid neutrals, pairing them with a different patterned piece
that repeats one of the other garment's base colors somewhere
on itself. If you're feeling particularly adventurous, plug in a
camouflage or leopard piece for extra credit. They are the wild
cards of the pattern-mixing master class—freaky enough to still
be edgy yet classically recognizable in their own way.

+ Pay attention to scale and size. An easy shortcut to mastering
pattern mixing is playing with scale. When you mix a larger print
with a smaller one, they have the effect of balancing one another
out—making one print the hero of the outfit story and the other
its loyal sidekick. I tend to think the larger print should be on the
bottom half of the outfit, as it grounds the look somewhat, but
I've also seen the opposite work, too—which is just further proof
that fashion rule makers don't always know what's best for you in
particular. All style advice should be taken with a grain of salt,
even when it's from me.

+ Always mix in a solid or neutral piece. A patterned shirt with a solid bottom and a contrasting, patterned shoe is an easy way to wear whatever the hell you want and still look office-appropriate. A neutral or solid piece can go a long way toward breaking up a too-fierce pattern mix. It also gives the eye a little relief from an overdose of visual excitement. If you need to tone down a pattern mix fast, classic navy is always your loyal, foolproof friend.

+ Test drive it first. Pattern mixing takes a certain amount of self-confidence, so make sure to road test your first attempts at it somewhere low impact—like for a day of running mindless errands. Your maiden pattern-mixing voyage shouldn't be anywhere high pressure like a wedding or school reunion. Wear it to the grocery store first—then, after someone compliments you on it, graduate to wearing it to work. It gets way easier every time you attempt it, I promise.

DUMB RULE NUMBER NINE: DON'T DOUBLE UP YOUR DENIM

Wearing denim-on-denim has been a solid fashion "don't" forever. But street style has blown right past that old idea, and it's now a totally cool fashion "do." However, there actually are a few rules to making it work.

This isn't a look for wallflowers. You'll need to make the whole point of your outfit the fact that yes, you are in fact boldly rocking denim on denim, and what of it? Don't be afraid to pair a pale blue, lightweight chambray shirt in a small repeating pattern with a pair of darker-wash boyfriend-style jeans. The trick is to mix the weights and shades of the denims you are wearing together. That way the look becomes all about contrasts in texture. Roll up your cuffs and finish the look with a pair of low-top white canvas sneakers and bare ankles. Two pieces of denim is really the max you should wear at any one time—but if you're feeling brave, you can match a pair of denim-accented kicks or a vintage jean handbag with your outfit and be the coolest kid in class.

DUMB RULE NUMBER TEN: REDHEADS CAN'T WEAR RED—AND BLONDES SHOULDN'T BE WEARING YELLOW, EITHER

The idea that your wardrobe can't echo your hair color is as anti-quated as the idea that blondes have more fun. But notice I said echo—not match—because to successfully pull off wearing a garment the same color as your hair, you'll need to choose a hue that flatters your locks instead of fighting them.

FOR REDHEADS

I once heard a snarky fashion commentator call a beautiful red-headed actor wearing a red dress a "walking valentine." I just rolled my eyes, because a redhead in the right shade of fiery red is a true thing of beauty, life, and vitality. The trick to a redhead wearing red successfully lies in finding a shade that is both richer and more intense than her hair:

+ Redheads whose hair is an orangey red should look for brighter blue-reds. (These colors look especially great with green or blue eyes.)

+ Redheads with hair in the brownish-auburn family should look for warmer, spicier reds that lean toward orange (including tomato red and paprika tones). The more brown the hair is, the more shades of red can be worn with ease.

+ Strawberry blondes look fabulous in clear, pinky reds but should avoid anything that has dusty overtones. Muddied colors have a tendency to look drab and dirty on pale redheads.

+ Coppery-toned redheads will get a lot of mileage out of true scarlet reds but should avoid any red that veers toward orange. Copper-colored hair already gives the look all the warmth it needs.

+ When wearing red, redheads should make sure to avoid higher-necked garments—they have a tendency to overpower the face with too high a dose of red-on-red goodness.

FOR BLONDES

Yellow is a color that automatically conjures up wholesome images of lazy summer afternoons and cheerful daydreams. Yellow is also a color that doesn't hog the spotlight and actually works quite well on blondes due to its inherently muted nature:

+ White or platinum blondes should look for bright sunshine and deep mustard hues but avoid pale yellow, which has a tendency to wash them out.

+ Champagne blondes can wear buttery yellow and lemon shades with ease but should pass on yellows that have an orange cast to them, because they tend to fight with the beige undertones champagne blondes naturally (or unnaturally!) have.

+ Butterscotch blondes can successfully wear almost any shade of clear yellow—but really pop in pineapple and taxi yellows.

+ Ashy blondes can pull off canary yellow and citron hues with surprising ease but should avoid wearing mustard yellow. It has a tendency to look drab next to hair with olive undertones.

+ All blondes can tone down a flat, blonde-on-yellow look by adding a piece in a color flattering to blondes into the mix. Navy and cognac both pair well with yellow and really make blonde hair pop.

Just because some boring nerd somewhere decided that we should all blindly follow a bunch of made-up fashion rules doesn't mean we have to obey. For every fashion "rule" ever written, there's just as compelling a reason to break them. So fly in the face of authority and carry on with your bad self, ya hear?

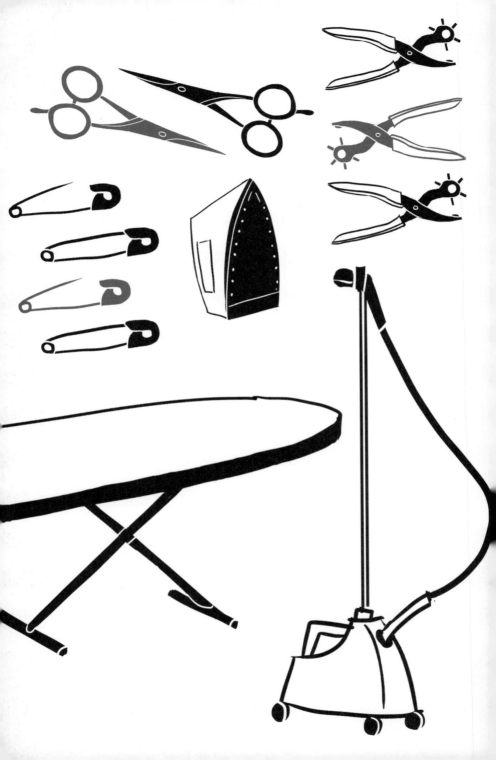

CHAPTER
6

WARDROBE
TOOLS
to keep your
look together

The thing that allows me to do my job better than anyone else on earth is my massive tool kit. I'm practically a carpenter of clothing, with gadgets and tricks for any wardrobe malfunction you could imagine. Actors don't just magically look good in their clothes without a lot of help—and producers don't want to hear my excuses when an actor realizes something is wrong with an outfit right before we are about to shoot. I've got to be able to fix any clothing-related disaster that could ever arise on the double—or risk being fired. You obviously don't need to own every single tool I use on set, but there are more than a few of them that you should consider keeping on hand to cut your own personal wardrobe malfunctions off at the pass.

Looking and feeling good in what you wear is all about putting in a little extra effort—and being adequately prepared will keep you and your clothes many steps ahead of everyone else. You could really boil the entirety of this book down to just that one central theme: Always. Be. Prepared. The time to solve a fashion disaster is before it happens, and that means having the tools you need already up your sleeve and ready to go. Everything I refer to in this chapter is available at my very favorite store on earth, Manhattan Wardrobe Supply (wardrobesupplies.com).

THE HOLY TRINITY:
SAFETY PINS, TOPSTICK, AND MOLESKIN

I have no choice but to lug an entire storage unit of stuff with me from show to show. But if I had to narrow it down to just three items, I know instantly what they would be—the holy trinity of wardrobe hacks: safety pins, Topstick toupee tape, and moleskin. With just these three items, you can fix almost any wardrobe tragedy right when it happens.

AND GOD CREATED SAFETY PINS
The humble safety pin is the hero of every story—because the number of wardrobe malfunctions you can solve with one is endless. The

modern safety pin is really just a piece of wire with a coil in the center that allows it to open up when released. It was patented in 1849 by a man named Walter Hunt, who then sold the patent for a measly four hundred bucks. Little did he know that its practicality would go on to make the new patent holder millions. At almost every fancy party I've ever been to, someone's dress strap has broken—necessitating a safety pin to fix it. (I once even repaired a hysterical bride's broken zipper with a fistful of safety pins I had stashed in my clutch moments before she walked down the aisle.) If you took the time to dump a handful of safety pins into the bottom of every purse you own right now, you'd pretty much be saving your own life. But a broken dress strap is only the beginning of its brilliant uses. Just by keeping a few different sizes of safety pins on hand, a girl really can rule the world.

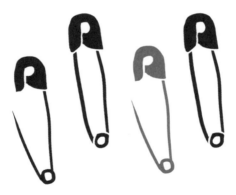

The Strapless Dilemma

Strapless dresses are my biggest nightmare—halfway through wearing one, it always starts to slide down, leaving my strapless bra hanging out. To avoid this phenomenon, I make sure to pin my bra to my dress, taking care to only grab the thinnest, innermost layer of the dress fabric so that the pin isn't visible from the outside of the garment.

The Emergency Zipper Pull

I own multiple jackets and sweatshirts that have been sporting a safety pin replacement zipper pull for years. It's simple, it works, and you can add a random charm to it for extra cuteness.

The Broken Shoe Strap

It's insane how even the most expensive pair of shoes can randomly snap a strap and leave you hobbling on the sidewalk. Keep a two-inch safety pin in your bag so you can hook it through the busted buckle and then stab it through the strap to get yourself back on the road.

Flip-Flop Blowouts

The classic flip-flop mechanism is a "T" style peg that pops into the hole in the sole and holds itself there. When you get a blowout and the peg will no longer stay in the hole, just guide the peg back into the hole and ram a safety pin through the bottom of it to mimic the "T." I speak from personal experience: this lazy fix will last you at least six months of heavy walking.

Keep Those Buttons Closed

You are probably all too familiar with being in the middle of talking to someone and suddenly realizing that half of your shirt buttons have popped open. For an easy fix, pin the space between each button closed with a miniature safety pin. With a little practice, you can master the art of grabbing only the tiniest bit or inside layer of the shirt fabric, rendering the safety pin unseen from the outside of the garment.

Master the "Instant Alteration"

It's amazing how many ill-fitting garments you can transform with a well-placed safety pin. My favorite trick is to gather a hunk of fabric at the back of the neck, fold it in a sort of "accordion pleat," and pin from the inside. Just like that, a top that was too big at the bust or under the arms is hiked up a few inches. Cover the pin with your hair and move on with your life.

Repair Jewelry on the Go

This is where it pays to have a few sizes of safety pins on hand in both gold and silver tones. If you have the right size pin, you can usually run it through the links of a broken chain to repair it and play it off as a style detail.

Restring a Hoodie

You can easily put a string back into a hoodie or pair of lounge pants using a simple safety pin. Just pin it through one end of the string and use the pin as a guide to work it back through the hole. I taught this trick to an actor who exclusively wore hoodies on a show, and he liked to give me heart palpitations by pulling the string out between takes and seeing how fast he could thread it back in before the director called "Action!"

Stop Static Cling

Simple safety pin science is the secret to keeping your tights from sticking to your skirt. Pinning a safety pin to the inside lining at the hem of your slip or skirt will conduct a small amount of static electricity and therefore help stop clinging. (A safety pin or two at a skirt's hem will also help weight down a hem that loves to flip up endlessly!) For more tips on how to fight static cling, flip to the Static Guard section on page 84.

Did you know that safety pins come in all sizes and colors? There are even solid black safety pins, which are way easier to hide in your clothes than the classic shiny silver ones. If you can't find them at your local sewing store (or are just feeling crafty), simply color the safety pins you already own black with a permanent marker. But a word of warning— color them before you use them on clothing—not once they are already in place.

BETTER LIVING THROUGH DOUBLE STICK TAPE

Did you ever wonder what held Jennifer Lopez's iconic jungle-green Versace dress in place at the Grammy awards way back in the year 2000? Viewers and fashion pundits were stunned at her plunging neck to navel display and kept themselves busy debating how on earth she was keeping it PG-13. I remember watching the awards and laughing the whole time, knowing exactly what she was using to pull off such a daring look—a few strips of double-stick toupee tape! (Yes, it's the same stuff bald dudes use.) I know how well it works, because I have applied copious amounts of it to some world-class breasts myself.

Medical grade toupee tape by Topstick is the gold standard, now and forever. However, in a pinch, regular old office supply double-sided tape does the job, too. I know this because that's what I brought to my first wardrobe gig. I was so green, I hadn't even heard of Topstick. It did the trick, and nobody ever even noticed. But don't be like me—get yourself a box of the original, used by wardrobe stylists the world over, available at Manhattan Wardrobe Supply for about $5.

How to Make a Skirt Behave

+ A spot of Topstick tape on your thigh keeps your skirt from flying up in an aggressive breeze. (Topstick uses medical-grade adhesive, so you can stick it to your skin without fear.)

+ Keep wrap dresses and skirts closed or in place with strategic Topstick placement.

+ Topstick your skirt to your undies to keep it from traveling around your body in an endless loop.

How to Hem Your Pants in Minutes

Use a piece of Topstick to create a fake hem in any garment. Iron it in place if you'd like, and press in a new crease where it belongs. Congrats, you've just hemmed your own pants or skirt in under five minutes. Sewing skills, who needs them? (Note: This is actually how I "hem" most of my actor's pants. But shhhh! Keep that factoid to yourself.) This hem will stay in place until you peel the Topstick off or wash it a few too many times.

Odds and Ends

+ Topstick is the perfect solution to tack down the ends of flopping belts.

+ A spot of Topstick also holds up thigh-highs and knee socks like nobody's business.

+ Keep your bra straps in place by sticking them to your garment with a dot of Topstick.

+ You can also use a piece of Topstick to help keep the gaps between buttons closed. But if you are rather large chested, this isn't your best solution—instead, use a handful of mini safety pins or have a tailor sew small plastic snaps (known as "babydoll" snaps) in between the buttons. They'll never pop open again!

Mastering Topstick Application

Topstick seems like a sticky mess until you master the technique of using it. Then it's easy as pie! You'll notice that one side of each piece has a small seam where the backing is in two pieces, while the other has a long, solid backing. Start by peeling the long, solid side off first, then sticking the exposed adhesive to your garment. After that, you can easily use a fingernail (or the pointy tip of a safety pin) to peel back each half of the perforated backing and let the top layer of the fabric you're attempting to adhere fall gently into place.

Topstick is surprisingly durable and stays put through numerous washings—but it can be peeled off with ease. When a piece of Topstick decides it's had enough, it simply removes itself from the garment in question and floats along in the washer like a bandage that's lost its stickiness. It doesn't tend to gum up your clothes up with leftover residue when you remove it, either. But leather belts are a different story—the adhesive can damage the finish if kept on for too long, so peel it off after every wearing and be sure to use a fresh piece the next day.

MARVELOUS MOLESKIN

Moleskin is a heavy cotton fabric that has been sheared on one side, giving it a short, cushy pile. It's a favorite of Brits and dandy dressers all over the world. But the type of moleskin I'm referring to here is actually coated with a sticky backing on the other side. It comes in handy sheets that you can cut to whatever size you need, and it's the perfect way to tame anything that rubs you the wrong way. You can find moleskin at any drugstore in the foot care aisle in both padded and flat versions. The padded kind provides blessed relief from heels that cut into your ankles and other such shoe problems, but you'll need to have the extra room in your shoe to accommodate it. I find the flat moleskin to be best for everyday use; it's endlessly customizable. I buy my moleskin for shows in bulk on a roll at Manhattan Wardrobe Supply—and they also carry it in black! The clothing, shoe, and accessory problems you can solve with a piece of moleskin and a pair of scissors are endless. My favorite fixes are below, but once you get your hands on a roll of moleskin, you're sure to come up with dozens of your own.

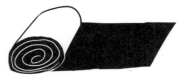

Shoes That Misbehave

Cut a piece to your desired size and use it to line anywhere inside a shoe that is cutting, digging, or rubbing your foot. Everyone thinks that moleskin is made to adhere to your skin—but I stick it right to the shoe itself. It's also the answer to sharp, skinny shoe straps that chafe and dig into the top of your foot. And moleskin is what I used to extricate myself from a disastrous situation when the offspring of two of the world's most famous actors started getting a blister due to the fancy leather shoes I put her in. Crisis averted, thanks to a spot of drugstore moleskin.

Bras That Claw

The clasps on my bras are always twisting around, causing the metal hooks to scrape right against my bare skin. Covering them with some moleskin trimmed to fit provides instant relief. You'll need to toss the old moleskin and cut a new piece to cover the hooks every time you wear that particular bra, unless you are a contortionist who is good at wriggling out of your bra without unclasping it. I precut a dozen or so pieces to the right size and keep them in my bra drawer for easy access.

Problem Jewelry

If your rings turn your fingers green, line the inside of them with a tiny strip of moleskin. If your problem is a ring that is a bit too big for your finger, just keep adding layers of moleskin in there until it fits.

Protruding Underwire

Fix your favorite bra by patching a protruding underwire with a small piece of moleskin. It'll hold the wire in place and keep it from poking you in the boobs. It also lasts through multiple wearings, as your body heat helps "set" the adhesive. When it finally gives up the ghost and loses its stickiness, just peel it off and pop on a new piece.

Scratchy Seams

If you have sensitive skin and end up cutting the tags out of every single garment you own, you'll love this. Use a custom-cut piece of moleskin to cover itchy, scratchy seams inside clothes, particularly the tail end of zippers on dresses. It's saved quite a few garments for me that I thought I'd have to give up on entirely.

EVEN MORE TOOLS TO KEEP YOUR LOOK TOGETHER

I'll go to my grave with a piece of moleskin, a handful of safety pins, and at least one strip of Topstick at the ready in my purse, but those are far from the only tools I use to keep my actors looking their best. Being prepared for any eventuality is what gets you ahead in life— and the same is true when it comes to maintaining your wardrobe.

BELT HOLE PUNCH

If you are still using the BBQ skewer or nail method to poke extra holes in your leather goods, I'll be visiting you in the hospital soon. I beg you, allow me to introduce you to a magical invention, one that I use almost daily: the belt hole punch.

This $20 tool solves more wardrobe problems than you even realized you had. Putting extra holes in belts is only the beginning. You can also alter the straps of shoes, book bags, and purses with this magical implement. I've even opened a beer bottle with mine in an "emergency." Tools that multitask: I love 'em.

PIT GUARDS

Armpit stains are one of the fastest ways to render a garment totally unwearable. And the sad, unhelpful solution to this problem is that it's best not to let it happen in the first place. I swear by the simplest invention ever—self-adhesive, stick-in armpit guards. They protect your dry-clean-only garments from ever even touching your sweaty armpits and run about $1 per pair. You'll make that money back almost instantly by not ruining your clothes and by stretching dry cleaning or laundering times between wearings. (You can also just cut a lowly panty liner in half and achieve the same effect for about twenty cents.) For a more permanent solution, look for actual fabric pin-in "dress shields" that can be removed and laundered frequently, available at most sewing and notions shops. They can be adhered by pinning, double stick taping, or stitching in place. If you decide to have them sewn in, ask your tailor to adhere them with tiny plastic snaps to make them easier to remove for laundering. Figuring out how to protect your garments from underarm stains in the first place is the single most valuable piece of advice in this book—or anywhere else, for that matter.

A MARKER THAT COULD SAVE YOUR LIFE

The humble black Sharpie is one of the most-used items in my wardrobe tool kit. It cheaply and instantly fixes scuffs on shoes and purses and is a great fake out for when you get a run in your opaque tights while you're out and about in the world. Just scribble the skin where the hole is and voila! It's camouflaged. (And, don't forget to replace those tights.)

LINT ROLLERS

It's amazing to me that people will go to the trouble to wear a really great outfit and then not invest two bucks in a lint roller to make sure they aren't dragging cat hair and random schmutz around on their backs all day. If you want to be of service to your extended family at a wedding or funeral, pack a mini lint roller in your suitcase. They will be flocking to your hotel room, I promise you. You can always make do with some tape rolled around your hand if you don't have a proper lint roller, but my money is on one of the sticky overnight shipping airbill pockets you may have lurking around your office. It makes a perfect makeshift de-linting device. Put it on like a mitt and pat the cat hair away.

PRE-THREADED NEEDLES

Every person reading this needs to take the time to learn how to sew on a button. But while knowing how to do so is a valuable life skill, threading a needle is a total waste of time. I use pre-threaded needles (available in a pack of ten in assorted basic colors from almost any sewing shop or drugstore) as often as possible, because what I don't need in my life is the tedious agony of trying to thread a needle in an emergency situation. It's total emancipation from ever having to squint into the eye of a needle like a cross-eyed wombat.

STATIC GUARD

I always use Static Guard brand antistatic, anticling spray when wearing layered clothes that love to stick to each other. I also spray my tights before putting a skirt on over them. The hair department on a show I worked on even taught me to spray a little Static Guard on my hairbrush to fight flyaways. In the winter, I spray the inside of my hat before putting it on to avoid staticky hat head later. In a pinch, you can also use a big squirt of regular old hair spray to fight static cling. But the very best, cheap, and cheerful static-fighting tip is to vigorously run a dryer sheet over whatever item is acting up. A single sheet lasts for at least twenty uses.

WET ONES

When an actor gets a stain on his or her costume, I reach for one stain remover before all others: Wet Ones antibacterial hand wipes. Available at your local drugstore for less than $3, they will remove almost any minor stain you could encounter as you go about your daily business. What makes them so good? It's the alcohol content in each wipe—it's not enough to damage most fabrics, but it gives a stain-removing boost regular wipes cannot. (For every single one of my stain-fighting secrets, flip to page 157.) Wet Ones are also the very best solution for removing deodorant marks from shirts. They don't shed bits of white fluff onto your clothes, making them a far better choice than regular baby wipes.

EXTRA SHARP EMBROIDERY SCISSORS

There are scissors, and then there are *scissors*. You haven't really lived until you've owned a deathly sharp pair of embroidery scissors small enough to snip the tiniest errant thread or poke out the eye of a Barbie doll.

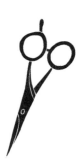

They are particularly brilliant if you hack the tags out of every garment like I do. The tips are severely pointed and allow you to cut with intense precision. You'll never accidentally put a hole in something because you were using a big, dull, clunky pair of scissors. In my opinion, there is no brand of scissors worth purchasing besides Gingher, available at better craft and fabric stores for anywhere from $10 to $50, depending on size.

NONSTICK COOKING SPRAY

Yes, I'm really talking about a can of classic nonstick cooking spray, available for about $3 at your local grocery store. This insane wardrobe fix was taught to me by one of the funniest actors working in Hollywood today. She must have broken a bunch of her toes at one point, because they were all sorts of mangled—making the high heels she had to wear in every single episode a nightmare to get into. Spraying her feet with a light coating of nonstick cooking spray allowed them to pop right into even the highest, tightest stilettos in a snap. I personally could not bear having my feet greased up like a suckling pig, but it really works, period. Actors know the darnedest things!

BUT WHAT ABOUT A BUSTED ZIPPER?

A busted dress zipper is never not a nightmare. And when it happens, there are sadly no good solutions. A zipper is really a mechanical instrument—so when it gives out, all hope is almost certainly lost. Your only options are either to have someone stitch you into the dress or close it up with a safety pin. (Of course, the one time it actually happened to me right before a wedding, I somehow had zero safety pins on hand. My best friend came to my hotel room, surveyed the situation, and said, "Well, at least it'll be dark soon.") Dresses with "invisible" zippers are the worst. The teeth of an invisible zipper are usually made of plastic and are notorious for bending, splitting, or breaking no matter how careful you are with them. All it takes is one extra ounce of pressure on the teeth as you zip past your ribcage, and suddenly the whole thing comes off the track, leaving you with nothing but a gaping expanse of skin and a sinking feeling in your heart. I don't even bother waiting for plastic zippers to break on set—because the odds of it eventually happening are too high. I replace them with metal separating zippers immediately. Metal teeth are far less likely to break because they are way sturdier than plastic.

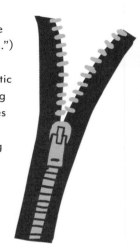

Since I am of the belief that it's not a question of if, but when a close-set invisible zipper snaps on you and ruins the event you were planning to attend, the only thing you can do to keep it from happening in the first place is to pay close attention when you zip your dress up. If at all possible, have another person do the actual zipping while you hold the sides of the zipper as close together as possible. When you don't take the time to hold the sides in order to help it slide more smoothly, you are putting excess pressure on the teeth—and subjecting them to possible bending.

In addition to recruiting a helper, you can also pretreat your zipper with a bit of soap or lip balm to help ensure a smooth zip. Never force a zipper if you can help it—most times, simply backing the zipper up and getting a "running start" will help it slide past the problem area with ease. Once a plastic zipper busts, don't waste your time trying to bend the teeth back into place—it's a fool's errand. On some metal zippers, you can carefully use a pair of tiny pliers to gently bend an errant tooth back into a functional position, but this is assuming you have a pair of tiny pliers on hand to begin with! Stitching the dress closed along the zipper track with a needle and thread (just to get you through the event—the zipper will eventually need to be replaced, of course) is sadly your very best option in this case. The key to making your temporary repair invisible is to use the strongest thread possible and work your way from top to bottom, using very small stiches.

If you can't get your hands on a needle and thread, let's hope you packed some safety pins. I like to use two sizes of pin to "repair" a busted zipper—a larger one-and-a-half or two-inch one for the pressure points (like at the widest part of the ribcage, the tail of the zipper, and the top) and a series of smaller pins to "stich" the rest of the zipper area closed.

As with any wardrobe malfunction, the best defense against a broken zipper is preparedness. So now that you've read this, you'll know to bring a spool of whatever thread matches your delicate party dress any time you travel—but it's also a good idea to tuck a tiny bar of soap, some mini pliers, and a handful of safety pins in your bag, too.

IRONING IS FOR SUCKERS

If you do only one thing from this book to improve your clothes, it's this: buy yourself a steamer. I am evangelical about the power of steam—because it's way too easy to ruin your clothes with an iron. Many delicate fabrics will shrivel, burn, and die when met with a hot iron—even on its lowest setting. That's not to say you should totally abandon your iron! There will always be a handful of garments that really do

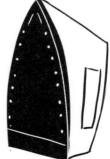

need a gentle pressing after hand washing, like pleated or intricately folded pieces. But a steady stream of steam will usually manage to coax even the most fragile garments back to life safely and effectively. Jiffy Steamer makes an old-school stand up steamer that will most likely outlive you, in addition to a travel-sized version that is all the steam you could ever need. My mentor gave me her 1970s-era full-size Jiffy when I first started in the business fifteen years ago, and it's still going strong. When I lost a wheel from dragging it through a parking lot at four in the morning, looking for a wardrobe trailer that hadn't yet arrived, I simply ordered a replacement wheel from the manufacturer. So if you ever find one at a garage sale in Hollywood, snap it up. Wardrobe girls have zero time for gear that can't take a beating.

A $20 chain-store steamer will definitely do the job at least half as well—but will most likely end up spitting water on your clothes. If this happens, cover the steam head with a sock, which will absorb any water droplets before they can get onto your clothes. (I like to use a sock meant for an infant—as turns out, a baby foot is about the same size as a steamer head!) To extend the life of any steamer you own, try to use only distilled water in it. This helps keep mineral deposits from crusting up the steamer, which is what causes it to spit water out onto your clothes in the first place. Also, here's a piece of obvious advice I had to figure out the hard way—don't steam your clothes when they are actually on your body. Steam is hot, and it will burn you.

IRONS ALSO COME IN CANS

If you still aren't sold on why you never need to touch an iron again, let me blow your mind and introduce you to the concept of an iron in a can—also known as wrinkle-releasing sprays. There are many commercially available ones on the market, but you can actually

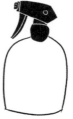

make your own by mixing one teaspoon of liquid fabric softener with one teaspoon of rubbing alcohol into one cup of distilled water (you can use regular tap water, but distilled water is always safer for your clothes because it doesn't contain minerals that could leave residue). Give it a good shake in a spray bottle that has a very fine spray nozzle, pull the garment taut, lightly spray the wrinkled area, and smooth the wrinkles out with your fingertips. It works on almost every single fabric and doesn't ever leave a stain. (One caveat: I'd test an inconspicuous area first before going full bore with it on something superdelicate like silk or chiffon.) Welcome to your new, completely iron-free life!

Wardrobe malfunctions are a sad fact of life that no amount of fame, money, or fancy clothes can prevent. But now that I've spilled every costume designer's secrets, tools, and tricks for solving them, keeping your look together is actually quite effortless. You just need to use the right tools!

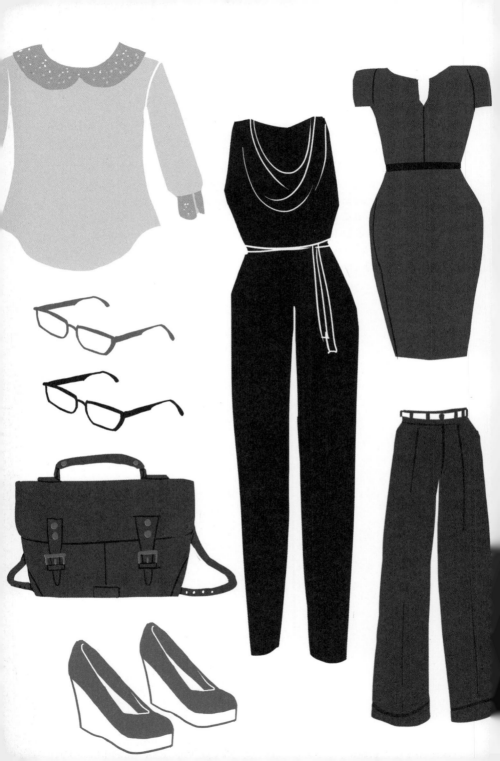

CHAPTER 7

DRESSING FOR SUCCESS IS DEAD

I often get asked, "What on earth do I wear to work or for a job interview?" and I always respond the exact same way: "Well, it depends on what type of job you want!" If you are pursuing a career as a dominatrix, I recommend a sturdy pair of five-inch spike-heeled boots (all the better to dig into a client's flesh with). And if your life dream is to be a waitress in a hot wings restaurant, I suggest learning your way around a pair of flesh-toned pantyhose and short shorts. If you've spent any time desperately looking for solid advice on what to wear in order to get ahead in life, you've probably read some version of the following recycled, unhelpful observations:

If you're wondering what to wear to an interview, the most important thing to keep in mind is that you must look professional and polished. While your interview attire depends on what job you're applying for, no matter what the position, you should come in looking neat, tidy, and appropriately dressed!

You don't say.

Being "appropriately" dressed at all times isn't just hard—it's boring, too. And what does "appropriate" even mean? It's highly subjective. While it's sadly true that people judge you by your clothes, I don't think they are judging you by the style of clothes you choose to wear—it's more likely that you are being judged for being lazy with what you wear.

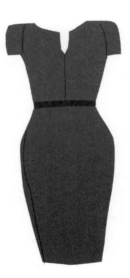

Allow me to explain.

I counsel every single person who asks me what to wear on a job interview to do some serious research as to what the general dress code of the job they're applying for is, and to then dress one level nicer than that. After all, you are technically a guest in their house—and looking to make a good impression! You can almost never go wrong with a suiting-quality skirt or trouser paired with a top that has some version of "buttons and a collar." If you're meant to wear a full business suit to the interview, it will be pretty obvious up front. It goes without saying that you must do a fingertip-length test of your skirt before leaving the house to make sure you can sit down in it without exposing your underwear. And, no, panty hose are not necessary anymore, unless you are interviewing at a law firm or in a similarly uberconservative field.

But none of this advice means that you have to whittle your personal style down to the typical and boring to be taken seriously at work. If your signature style veers toward a rockabilly or goth vibe, you should by all means wear red lipstick and victory rolls or Victorian-inspired ankle boots with your proper skirt suit. Sometimes pure personality is the thing that separates you from others who can do a job just as well as you. Your style is part of what makes you special and memorable.

But the devil of dressing to impress really is in the details. For example, being a costume designer doesn't just mean I'm responsible for dressing the stars in expensive, custom-made ensembles. Every single show also has at least two to two hundred extras or "background actors." These are the folks who fill up bars, law offices, and hospital waiting rooms so our lead actors don't appear to be the only ones existing on Planet Earth. These extras almost always bring their own wardrobe, and it's up to the costume department to dig through their options and assign something appropriate from the choices they present to us. Without fail, there is always one person whose clothes are obviously inexpensive pieces from a discount store or are even secondhand, but that are maintained and kept up impeccably. This person's look always trumps someone with more expensive pieces that haven't been treated very well.

A $20 blazer from a thrift store that has been pressed, repaired, and tailored to fit the wearer will *always* look far better than a $200 blazer that reeks of smoke and has been crammed in the trunk of a car for two weeks—because proper wardrobe maintenance is the true cornerstone of "dressing for success." Before you leave the house for any occasion, but specifically for a job interview or similarly important event, you should be asking yourself six very important questions:

ARE MY CLOTHES DIRTY?

This sounds crazy obvious, but it bears repeating. Dirty, stained clothes are doing your appearance no favors—and you can be sure that people are noticing. (You don't want to be the "woman with the stain" when interviewers are sorting through applicants.) Dry cleaning bills add up fast, but knowing how to care for your dry-clean-only garments at home can cut costs immensely and allow you to stretch time between cleanings drastically. (Find out more about this witchcraft in chapter 10!) Not every garment needs to be cleaned after every single wearing—and excessive exposure to dry-cleaning fluid can cause a garment's fibers to become brittle and dry, thereby wearing out the garment faster.

In most cases, simply hanging your garment in a well-ventilated spot between wearings will allow odors caused by smoke or food to fade. Invest in a large, soft-bristle brush (like a shoe-shine brush) to spot-clean any bits of food or grime that are sitting on top of the garment's fibers. Start by going against the grain of the cloth using short, quick strokes. Finish off with a second light brushing that goes with the nap, returning it to its former glory. If you spill greasy food or drink on your garment, spot clean it as gently as possible—preferably by blotting the fabric with clean water and a cloth rag. (This works best on wool or cotton fabrics.) Stains on light-colored or silk fabrics require quick attention and should be hand washed or taken to the cleaners as soon as possible. Avoid home remedies such as club soda and salt—and never rub a stain or put water on any fabric that can't be washed in water; you're likely to damage it and leave a ring. Blotting with a clean cotton cloth is your very best bet if you are unsure. (And for more info on fighting stains, flip to page 157.) In between dry cleanings, you can also refresh your garments with an at-home dry-cleaning system. They are great for removing slight odors and general refreshing, but are not meant to be a replacement for proper dry cleaning.

There is really no hard and fast timetable as to how often your garments need to be cleaned—unless we are talking about garments you are putting away for the season. Winter coats, summer dresses, and other season-specific pieces need a cleaning after months of hard wearing and before being stored for any period of time.

ARE MY CLOTHES WRINKLED?

Wrinkled clothes are a clear sign to the world that you don't really care about your look. Taking an extra five minutes to straighten things out is well worth the time investment. But as we discussed on page 87, you don't even need to own an iron to keep your clothes unwrinkled. Not only is using a steamer far easier than ironing, it also removes faint odors and freshens garments between wearings. I pack my travel steamer whenever I'm traveling for a wedding, and there is inevitably a line of people outside my hotel room door in the hours before the ceremony—sometimes even the bride herself!

AM I SHOWING SOMETHING I WISH I WASN'T?

The wisdom goes that women looking to be taken "seriously" as "professionals" should take great care to avoid anything too low cut, sheer, or revealing. That makes sense on the face of it, but doesn't take into account that some women with big boobs or bangin' booty curves can never wear *anything* without it being revealing—no matter how hard they try. I can't help you tone down your lovely bum shape (and why would you want to?), but you can easily avoid showing more cleavage than you intended with a simple closet of old-school camisoles.

They cleverly fill in the gap on a low-cut blouse, render a sheer top totally office-appropriate, and add coverage and length to a top that tends to ride up. It's a rare day that I don't have one on underneath whatever I happen to be wearing. A good closet of camisoles includes both silky, lacy options that are meant to be seen peeking out of your blouse and simpler, seamless, spandex-infused versions that provide maximum coverage. Your work wardrobe isn't complete without them, and chances are good that you're revealing more than you really want to if you're not wearing one.

ARE MY CLOTHES COVERED IN LINT, PILLS, OR STRAY THREADS?

Before you leave the house every day, take the time to run a masking tape–style lint roller over your outfit. Random cat hair and household schmutz clinging to your clothes is the opposite of professional and put together. Stray threads are another huge look-killer that can easily be slayed by keeping a mini pair of scissors handy in your dresser drawer. Paying close attention to these two things alone will elevate your work look from sloppy to sassy almost instantly.

Pilling is what happens when fibers ball up on a garment after washing or wearing, creating unsightly little bobbles hanging off your clothes. They are especially common on areas that receive a lot of friction. Synthetic fabrics are particularly bad at pilling because they are stronger than natural fabrics (such as wool, silk, or linen) so any pills that do form hold on for dear life. Pills are bad news, because they make you look like you don't care about how you're presenting yourself to the world. Luckily they are one of the easiest wardrobe problems to solve! I use either a $1 disposable razor or a $3 device called the D-Fuzz-It to "shave" pills off garments effortlessly. For less than four bucks, you can keep your clothes looking brand new at all times—even if they're really not.

ARE MY SHOES SCUFFED, DIRTY, OR WORN?

Whenever I meet someone, I always notice the state of his or her shoes. You might think that means I'm a big 'ol snob, but shoes (not the eyes, where'd you hear that?) really are the windows of the soul. Proper shoe shines are not just for the boys of the *Mad Men* era, either. Anyone looking to be taken seriously in their profession can benefit from the regular buffing, polishing, and cleaning of their footwear. How your shoes look really does matter! My dad taught me how to shine my own shoes when I was about seven years old. Sure, you can take your shoes to a cobbler for a little TLC, but nothing beats doing it yourself. (Skip to page 172 for my dad's tried-and-true spit-shine steps.) If you wear high heels regularly, be sure to keep an eye on the very tips of your heels as they wear down shockingly fast and when worn down can cause permanent damage to the heel. You can buy replacement tips from most places that sell shoelaces and easily tap them into place with a hammer for an instant do-it-yourself fix.

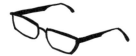

DOES THIS FIT ME PROPERLY?

Are your pants too long? Do your hems drag on the ground, tripping you up and getting dirty and frayed in the process? Do your shirts gap at the buttons and flash your bra when you don't intend to? Are you swimming in a size large, yet a size medium is too small for you? If so, your look is suffering severely from lack of clothes that fit properly—and proper fit is the number one thing that can take a look from slovenly to sharp in ten seconds flat.

We covered the basics of proper fit way back in chapter 2 (which seems so long ago now!), but it bears repeating here as well. Finding the pieces that suit you and making them part of your go-to style helps you look your best at work or in any other professional situation. I'll also never stop banging the drum about alterations, because they are insanely important. So you're going to hear me say it over and over again: the main reason movie stars look like movie stars in their clothes is because of simple alterations. Almost no garment fits anyone correctly right off the rack. A few bucks on an alteration here and there makes a huge difference as to how a garment fits you and how you then look to the world. I have never, ever, not even once in my career put an actor on camera in an article of clothing that hasn't had at least one alteration—no matter how small.

You can find my cheat sheet of the simple (yet life-changing) alterations I do for every single actor I ever dressed back in chapter 3. Most of them will cost you less than twenty bucks at your local dry cleaner—yet give you ten times that value in return.

The real truth of "dressing for success" is that sometimes, the trick to looking better in your clothes is simply to have fewer of them. While that sounds confusing, it's really not! We've been conditioned to think that to look good all the time, we need an endless supply of clothes so as never to be seen in the same thing twice—but in fact, the opposite is true. It's far better to have fewer clothes that are of better quality than an avalanche of clothes that aren't so great. When I see someone who wears a truly great suit once every single week like clockwork, I never think, "Ugh, why is she or he wearing that again?" Every time, I just think, "Man, that really is a fabulous friggin' suit." Simply paying a little extra attention to the condition of what you're wearing elevates your look far more than a closet bursting with poorly cared-for clothes ever could. So wear your favorites as often as you like. Because honestly, absolutely nobody is judging you—unless your favorites just so happen to be covered with cat hair and coffee stains.

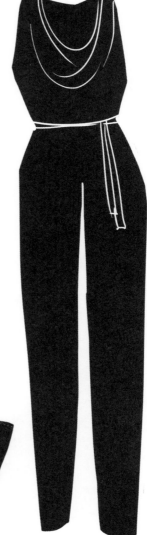

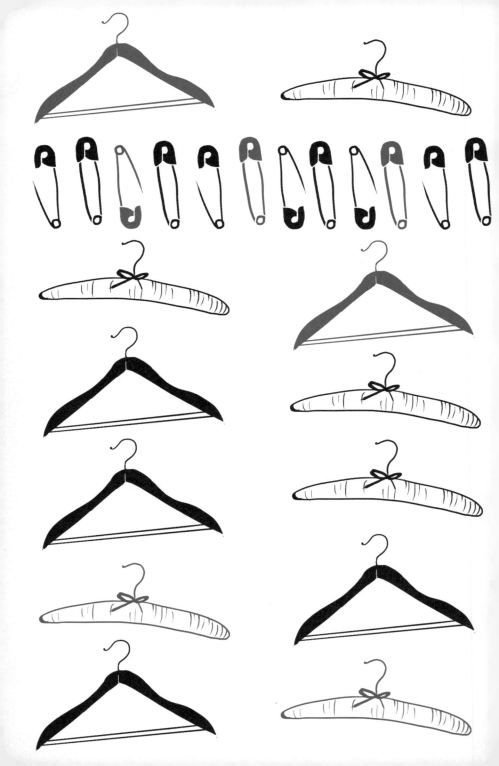

CHAPTER 8

CLOSET HACKS:
store your clothes like wardrobe girls do

Working on set is a life like no other—if you can learn to take the heat. There's zero margin for error on a production, and nobody cares what your problems and excuses are. You have to be able to put your hands on whatever you need to do your job at the exact second you realize you need it. Organization is not optional—it's the difference between life and death.

My personal closet at home is all things to all people. It's both a magical wonderland, where pals can come to borrow party dresses, and a living, breathing nightmare to those who fear clutter. I'm not too concerned—because it somehow works for me, and I love digging through my mess! I continually find things in my closet that surprise me—and that I have no recollection of ever even acquiring. It makes for a great mystery every morning when I go to get dressed, because I never know what I'm going to get! But trust me, it's no way to live.

WHEN IN DOUBT, JUST HANG IT UP!

My actor's closets on set are another story entirely. They are organized like you wouldn't believe—because my entire job depends on being able to find whatever I need in seconds flat while 150 extras are milling about in period costumes, the star actor is off the clock in twenty minutes, no exceptions, and someone is screaming hysterically in my ear that they need it now, now, now! You'd be pretty unpleasantly surprised to learn how easy it is for an actor to lose an earring, break a shoe strap, realize their bra hurts, or decide they actually do need a belt with those pants (even though you asked them a thousand times if they needed one in the fitting).

To be ready for anything a production can throw at me, I use a simple yet magnificent way to keep everything close at hand, right where I could see it for easy access yet still make good use of my limited space on stage. While this sounds like a crazy luxury only available in glamorous Hollywood, it's really not. You can make your own closet just as streamlined, functional, and organized as the stars' closets are by utilizing every costumer's secret organizational weapon. It's both ridiculously easy and totally revolutionary. Ready?

Just hang everything up.

The only things I don't store on hangers in my actor's closets are shoes and handbags. Hanging storage solutions do exist for those items, but I think they are way too bulky and take up valuable rail space. I prefer to store handbags in plain old plastic laundry baskets and cover every door in sight with hanging shoe racks. Just put your fanciest shoes on the side of the door that the whole world can see—it's instant art!

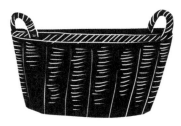

But yes, I do indeed hang up all my actor's clothes, bras, jewelry, underwear, belts, scarves, accessories, and even tights and stockings. And you should, too—because if you can't clearly see it, you aren't ever going to wear it. Drawers are for suckers—and hiding ratty old gym clothes. (However, don't worry if you don't have enough rail space to hang everything up; there are ways to work around it on page 109.)

START WITH THE RIGHT HANGERS—AND HANG YOUR STUFF UP RIGHT

For shirts, dresses, and blouses—really anything that can be hung on regular hangers—I am evangelic about investing in a set of slim line, flocked "velvet" hangers. Not only do they maximize your rail space like crazy, they also usually have a small hook on one side so you can cascade hangers and garments down, one after the other, utilizing the wasted space that always exists below your short garments. But if you don't want to spring for new hangers, you can get the same effect with the hangers you already own by using old soda can tabs. They are free and have two sturdy openings, making them perfect for the job! Just slip one around the hook of the hanger you already have on the rail, and then offset your next hanger through the second opening. This tip only works with thinner, metal-hooked hangers, not thick plastic ones. And have no fear—the modern-day pull-tab is designed to have zero sharp edges that could snag your clothing. So if you take nothing else from this chapter, let it be this: utilizing every single inch of available vertical space is the name of the game when it comes to wardrobe storage.

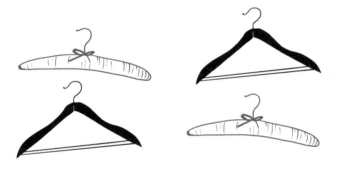

While hanging your clothes up sounds totally easy, there's a really good chance you are hanging up some of your favorite garments all wrong. Sweaters in particular have a terrible tendency to slide off a hanger at the slightest provocation, not to mention that hanging delicate knits can stretch them out and cause "shoulder nipples." So instead of hanging a sweater the same way you would any old shirt, just lay it flat on a table, fold in half lengthwise (making sure the armpits and cuffs match up), and fold it around the hook part of the hanger—making sure all the weight is now centered in the armpit of the folded sweater at the top of the hanger where the hook is. Then fold the arms and the bottom half of the sweater around the hanger. This sweater will now never, ever slide off of a hanger again.

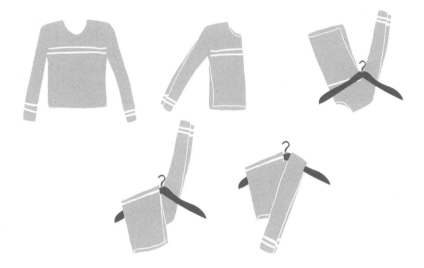

Sadly, I learned how to hang a sweater like this the hard way. Once upon a time, I was but a lowly wardrobe assistant, tasked with returning a rack of fancy clothes to a swanky Beverly Hills department store. One of the items was a nearly $900 cashmere sweater, which I neatly hung on a hanger like any normal person would—the way I'd been doing my entire life, and likely the way you're hanging sweaters right now! However, as I rolled the rack of clothes across the parking lot, that sneaky cashmere sweater slipped right off the hanger and got caught up in the wheel of the rack, becoming black, filthy, and covered with oil in the process. Of course this sweater could no longer be returned to the store, and would you like to take a guess as to who ended up paying for it?

I gave my employer $50 out of my paycheck every single week like clockwork until I had finally paid for the entire thing. I threw that stupid sweater in the trash the minute I made the last "payment" and never looked back. But as my mother always says: "A bought lesson is better than a taught one." There really is no wardrobe disaster that hasn't already happened to me, and there's as much to be learned from my mistakes as there is from my years of experience.

I hang as many pants and skirts as I can by folding them over the bar of a regular hanger, but a handful of proper clip hangers are a necessity for certain pieces that just won't stay on a bar hanger. You can buy special clip accessories that turn those fancy velvet hangers I love so much into clip hangers, but if you're looking to economize, just do what I do— use old-school clothespins to make a shirt hanger into a skirt hanger. They are about two bucks for three dozen and work like a charm.

If you use clip-style clip hangers in your closet, protect the waistband of your delicate skirts and pants from hanger indentations by slipping a bit of tissue paper (or even just actual bathroom tissue!) between the clip and your garment. I hoard the tissue that comes in shoeboxes for this exact purpose.

HANGERS ARE MEANT FOR MORE THAN JUST CLOTHES

Despite what Mommie Dearest had to say about wire hangers, I use them in every closet I am in charge of—but never for hanging up clothes! You should definitely switch those wire hangers out for proper hangers the very minute your garments come home from the dry cleaners, as they are not meant for long-term storage. I "recycle" all my paper-covered wire hangers by converting them into jewelry, scarf, and stocking holders—I even use paper hangers to store bras and underwear! This is the real benefit of hanging up everything you own in plain sight—because with a stash of free paper hangers from the dry cleaner and a handful of safety pins, and you'll never need to spend money on a proper organizing device again.

I know what you're thinking: "Wait a minute. Everything? You mean I should hang up my bras and underwear too?"

Yep, that's right—you can finally get your lingerie drawer under control simply by removing the drawer from the equation. Your bras, underwear, stockings, slips, and tights will be way more organized if you store them on hangers. Just pass the straps of each bra through a safety pin (taking care not to pierce through the strap itself if you can help it) and then pin them in a row across a paper hanger, starting at the middle and working your way out toward each side to help balance the weight. It takes a little longer to remove and replace them, but it's well worth it.

You can't imagine how much time this little "bra tree" saves you every morning when you don't have to dig in a deep, dark drawer for a specific bra to wear with a certain blouse. (Plus, it saves your bras from being crushed to death by being stored on top of each other.) For strapless and other convoluted styles, I either slip a smaller pin through the tag or hook and eye closure—or find the least damaging spot to pin into. I've stored thousands of dollars of bras and other lingerie in this manner without incident, so have no fear. If I have a matched set of bra and panties, I pin them right next to each other on the hanger so I remember to wear them together. You can also hang tights, slips, and stockings in the same manner, making sure to always pin through the thickest part of the waistband.

What else can you store on a lowly paper hanger? Just about anything you can stick a pin through: scarves, jewelry, belts, accessories—basically anything you reach for daily and can't always find easily. It's my favorite storage tip there ever was. I'd suggest grouping like items together on one hanger, as it helps immensely when you're trying to determine what accessory to pair with what you're wearing. It allows you to pull out an entire hanger of belts (or scarves, or tights) and hold each one up to your outfit without digging around in your closet like a deranged rat scrounging for something to hold up your pants.

If you don't have an endless supply of paper hangers on hand because you don't do much dry-cleaning (and you really shouldn't be dry cleaning most of your clothes—jump ahead to chapter 10 to read all about how to skip the dry cleaner completely), you can just use one of Hollywood's very best secret organizational tricks—the muslin hanger. Available for about $13 each at Manhattan Wardrobe Supply, these sturdy, curved wooden hangers are covered on both sides with a 12-inch square of natural muslin fabric and will easily replace every single scarf, belt, tie, jewelry, or bra organizer your local big-box store has to offer. All you need to get organized with one is a handful of safety pins! Muslin hangers take up far less space than most organizing gadgets and can be used to store exactly everything you own. A muslin hanger covered with dozens of beautiful scarves can even become a work of art, ready for hanging on a random doorknob or wall hook.

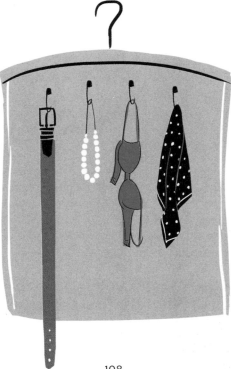

If your scarves are too heavy or delicate to hang with a pin, just slip them into a clear sandwich bag and then pin that onto your paper or muslin hanger. I store everything in my on-set closets in see-through bags—because if you can't easily see it, you won't remember that it's there. (And, again, you're less likely to wear it!) When it comes to hanging up your entire closet, your wicked imagination (and possibly your rail space) is the only thing stopping you.

After reading this, you might be wondering where on earth you'd store all those blasted safety pins for easy access. Well, this one's easy. Get your paws on the low-tech device your grandmothers (and their grandmothers!) have used for centuries: an inexpensive hanging clothespin bag. Hang one at the end of your closet rail and fill it with safety pins so you can be a nonstop accessory-storing machine. (Alternatively, if you have a bit of extra countertop space, you could repurpose a magnetic paperclip holder to corral your mess of safety pins for easy access. I use one for my bobby pins in the bathroom too!)

BUT WHAT IF I DON'T HAVE ENOUGH RAIL SPACE?

If you don't want to (or can't) hang up everything you own due to space, there are still a bunch of clever ways that you may not have considered to make your closet work better. Here are some of my favorite storage ideas (both from work and home!):

DRAWERS: If you have a lot of jewelry, repurpose a few of your dresser drawers into a bauble armoire using cheap cutlery or ice cube trays from the supermarket. Dedicate one tray to earrings, another for bracelets, and so on. It's much easier to see and wear all of your jewelry when it's spread out rather than crammed into a tiny jewelry box. If you don't own enough jewelry to need entire drawers in which to store it, do what I do when I need to make my jewelry kit mobile on a location shoot— use either a plastic tool box (the kind with a handle) or a fishing tackle box. All the varied compartment sizes make it practically impossible to be disorganized.

PEGBOARD: You can also utilize an old-school pegboard and hooks to store jewelry as art on an unused wall. (This is how they do it at the costume house, by the way.) It's life changing to have your entire jewelry collection neatly hung before your very eyes. You can also adapt this idea to utilize the space inside of bathroom cabinets and armoire doors.

CARDBOARD TUBES: Start stockpiling old toilet paper and paper towel tubes to store your tights and stockings in. Sound insane? Not once you use a marker to write on the outside of the tube and carefully roll your legwear up inside. Now you can see what you have at a glance, and your stockings are neatly organized and tangle-free—all for zero dollars. Once you've crammed your clean (or not-so-clean, who am I to judge) legwear into their labeled tubes, you can toss them into a drawer or bin without thinking twice about organization—because they practically organize themselves. It's both totally neurotic yet incredibly lazy at the exact same time, making it my very favorite type of organizational hack.

BOOKSHELVES: If your shoe habit is totally out of control, consider turning the pairs that won't fit inside your closet into conversation pieces by repurposing an old bookshelf into a miniature shoe parlor. When I did this at my old apartment, I made it a full-fledged display by putting tchotchkes and found objects in between all the shoes. This works best with your prettiest pairs—so keep those ratty workout sneakers under the bed where they belong. (I stash all my unsightly gym shoes in cardboard wine boxes I get for free from the supermarket. They're actually perfect, because they already have built in dividers!)

POOL NOODLES, NEWSPAPER, AND WINE BOTTLES: Tall boots are always a pain to store—as the tops flop over and make them a nuisance unless you invest in expensive boot stays for every single pair. But you can make your own for free just by stuffing your boots with newspaper. Not only does it keep them upright, newspaper helps absorb the sweat and odors your boots pick up when you wear them all day, every day. If you're not a newspaper subscriber, try hacking up a pool noodle (those cylindrical foam things kids are always playing with at the pool, available anywhere that sells beach gear) to fit the height of each boot. They'll never tip over again. I cut mine using a serrated bread knife and a cutting board, and you should be able to do two or three pairs of boots with each noodle. (Alternatively, you can just use an empty wine bottle in each boot to keep 'em upright!)

TIE RACK: I wear camisoles or tank tops under almost everything I own—so my collection of them is quite large. Instead of hanging every single one on a separate hanger, I enlisted a cheapo men's tie rack into service to hold them all. It takes up very little closet space and holds over twenty-five tank tops.

BUTTONS: If you are forever losing a pair of tiny earrings, consider storing them with the posts threaded through the holes of a spare button. It keeps pairs together—and ensures you'll never be scrambling for a missing earring back when you're in a hurry.

SHOWER CURTAIN RINGS/HOOKS: If you can spare the rail space, one of the best ways to store handbags, scarves, or belts is using something you likely have on hand already: shower curtain rings or hooks! Whether you hang them from the bottom bar of a wooden hanger or right onto your closet rail, they keep everything front and center, right where you can see it—and wear it.

WARDROBE RACK: If you don't have a closet at all, don't fret! Just turn a corner of your bedroom or living room into your own personal *atelier* (that's French for a designer's workshop or studio) by utilizing a pro-style chrome wardrobe rack with a wire bottom shelf and calling attention to your excellent taste in clothes and shoes. I love clothes out in plain sight—as they immediately become a point of interest in your home. (But then, I believe that clothes are a form of art.) You can also DIY a bottom shelf for your wardrobe rack by having an inexpensive piece of plywood cut to fit at your local lumber store, and you can store almost everything you own in one neat package. I also spray paint plain old plastic laundry baskets fun colors to give them a little pizazz and to have a place to store all my handbags and shoes. (And PS: Don't waste your money on a cheap, flimsy white metal rack from a big-box store—it'll bend and break on you after barely any use. Those bright, shiny polished chrome rolling racks that retail for between $50-$69 are the very ones professional wardrobe stylists and costume designers use—they last forever, and replacement parts for them are easy to find. So accept no substitutes!)

FABRIC GARMENT BAGS: Storing out-of-season clothes is a good way to save space, but you can't just put everything in a trash bag and shove it in the attic. Fabric has a tendency to degrade faster than you might think, so take the time to store your off-season pieces right. First things first: Make sure anything you are putting away for an extended period of time is clean and dry. Sweat and body oils can attract bugs, and even slight stains will permanently set themselves if left too long. Never hang clothing you are planning to store for an extended period of time—especially knit items. The pressure can cause shoulders to fray and the entire garment to become misshapen. Items that are being stored should be folded and stacked loosely, keeping heavier items on bottom. This allows air to keep circulating around the clothes— thereby avoiding mold and mildew. If you must keep special-occasion items on hangers, use a wide-arm suit jacket hanger to spread the weight more evenly on the garment. And don't zip them up tight in plastic garment bags—look for fabric versions that protect your garments from light and dust while allowing air to move in and out freely. If you can't find (or just don't want to pay for) fabric garment bags, an old pillowcase with a slit cut in the top for the hanger to poke through is a great, cheap alternative. We buy them in bulk at thrift stores when storing a show's wardrobe at the end of a season for this exact purpose!

SUITCASES: Plastic containers are a good choice for temporary clothing storage when kept in a strict temperature-controlled environment, as they stop moths in their tracks—but any moisture trapped inside a sealed container will eventually create its own microclimate and lead to mold and mildew settling in. An old suitcase that has been cleaned and lined with acid free tissue (available at most art supply stores) is one of the best storage containers there is. Never use plastic from the dry cleaner to store clothes; again, plastic does not allow air to circulate freely and leads to mold and rot. If you don't have a suitcase to spare, you can either drill a few holes in a snap-lid plastic bin or look for one that has a nonairtight flip-top lid. Mothballs and cedar can be used as insurance against moths—but neither is a guarantee that you won't still end up with holes in your clothes.

The best place to store your tissue-lined suitcase (loosely packed with clean, folded clothes!) is in a cool, dry, dark place. Light, heat, and dampness are the triple enemies of clothing—making an attic or basement a less than ideal spot to store them. Once your garments are stored, don't forget about them! Check both the outside of your containers and what's being stored inside regularly so you can nip problems in the bud—and be sure to give anything that's been stored for a year or more a wash before wearing it again to remove any small stains that may have cropped up while they were taking a break.

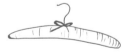

The same old dumb pearl of "wisdom" gets trotted out during any discussion about closet organization: "You should regularly purge your closet of things you haven't worn in six months to a year!" While there *is* sometimes such a thing as having too many useless clothes, don't just blindly follow this overly simplistic platitude, because you're likely going to need whatever you tossed for a costume party one day and end up being very sorry. (The only exception to this rule is stuff that doesn't fit and you don't feel great in. Say goodbye to all that and never look back, no matter how much those items originally cost.) But when you store your clothes like wardrobe girls do, what you should keep and what you should toss becomes totally obvious—because it's right there in front of your eyes. See how easy that was?

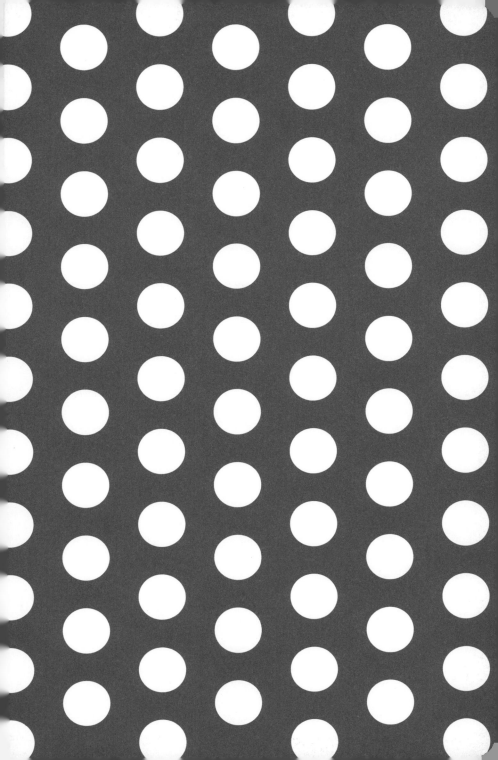

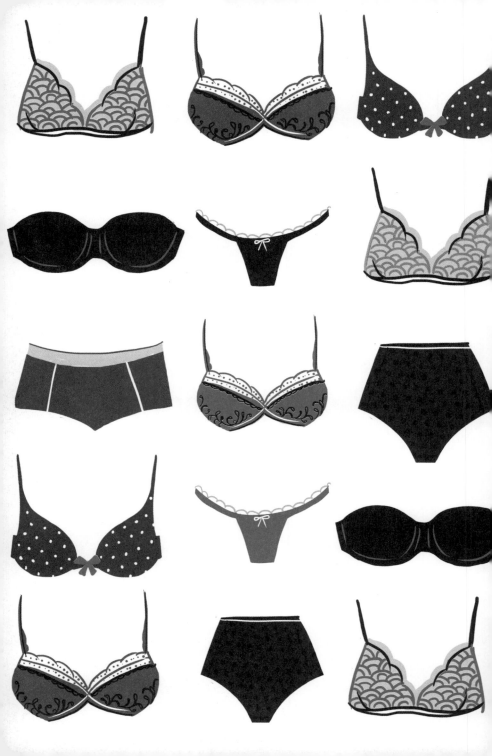

—

CHAPTER 9

UNDERTHINGS:
*you really only
need a few*

Undergarments are a pretty ridiculous concept, if you really think about it. Why are we meant to wear a special set of clothes underneath our regular clothes? (I guess for, like, sanitary reasons and stuff?) I'm not saying that I think you should go without undergarments, but I do happen to think that everything you thought you knew about bras, slips, and underwear is actually wrong, wrong, wrong (but especially about bras).

FIRST THINGS FIRST: THROW YOUR SHAPEWEAR IN THE TRASH

I am pretty staunchly anti-shapewear, at least when it's used to make one look "skinnier." Because it really doesn't! Sausage still looks like sausage, even when it's in a casing. The whole idea of these horrifically constricting undergarments being necessary is a giant, cruel joke that we've all been happily seduced into spending millions upon millions of dollars on. The actors I dress regularly show up to fittings with their own personal undergarment "rig"—a frighteningly restrictive amount of spandex and Lycra meant to squeeze, tuck, mold, and reshape their natural assets into whatever Hollywood is currently deeming "acceptable."

I put actors (both male and female!) in a modified version of shapewear for only two reasons—smoothing and coverage. Smoothing as in not having any bulky, lumpy seams visible under clothes, and coverage as in having their lovely cheeks remain covered, should they find themselves with skirts suddenly up over their heads. When I really do need to put someone in a sleek, long-legged control garment,

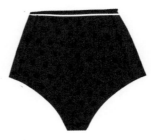

I always buy a size up from what the size chart suggests in order to avoid death by slow lower-body asphyxiation.

You may be surprised to learn that I hit up the lingerie departments of discount and department stores for old-school girdles and cute granny panties instead of blowing my cash on name-brand "slimming" shapewear. Because despite what you may have heard, the idea that granny panties are some horrible, shapeless, floral cotton things that only unsexy women wear is totally false. The classic 1950s style high-waist panty is easily one of the sexiest lingerie looks going! Its lines echo the natural shape and folds of the body and provide a long, smooth, uninterrupted line underneath clothes. The full bottom coverage is extremely coquettish and comes in quite handy if you encounter a giant gust of wind or just happen to be a bit unladylike when you sit or bend over.

My other secret shapewear substitute is a plain old pair of cotton or microfiber bike shorts. They cover all the bases—protecting thighs from rubbing themselves raw due to chafing (sometimes known as "chub rub"), protecting cheeks from possible prying eyes, and stopping panty lines in their tracks. They are at least twenty times more comfortable than traditional control garments, and a pair of lace-trimmed bike shorts can also look ridiculously cute peeking out from the hem of a skirt or dress. But beware the waistband and front seam on most bike shorts, which will show like crazy underneath a sheer or tight skirt.

Both granny panties and bike shorts manage the job of covering your lady-bits for less money than traditional shapewear—and without stopping the flow of blood to your lower extremities or rolling down around your waist like a cartoon window shade that's about to cut you in half. And best of all, you aren't forced to pee out of a small hole as with most shaper garments—which is a shameful experience, no matter how you try to spin it. I was once part of a costume crew tasked with taking care of a big-name actor who loved to wear a full-body shaper suit at all times. Every single time she had to use the bathroom,

HOW TO GET DRESSED

it was a huge, dramatic production that I had to help with. Fourteen hours into an eighteen-hour day, said actor nonchalantly announced to me from the other side of the bathroom door that she had accidentally wet herself—and could I please have someone bring her backup bodysuit from the wardrobe trailer?

The trailer was an incredibly inconvenient, fifteen-minute van ride away. I dutifully sounded the alarm and got word within minutes that a costumer was already on the road, burning rubber toward the set with the spare bodysuit. In the meantime, I had the entire production hysterically freaking out on me over the walkie-talkie headset I had jammed into my ear, wondering where in the hell their star was. I put them off and made excuses until I could no longer stand it—at which point I politely excused myself from the bathroom, stepped outside, and calmly announced to the entire production over a wide-open walkie channel: "She pissed herself, okay? I'm doing the best I can." The line was silent for almost a full minute until finally our assistant director came on and said, "Copy that! Let me know when you're all cleaned up."

The moral of this story is not to find yourself in this situation in the first place—because when peeing through a hole goes south in the real world, you're not going to have a fancy Hollywood costume designer at your side to help. You'll be stuck cramming your urine-soaked shapewear garment into your handbag and slinking home.

DON'T FEAR THE PANTY LINE

Panty lines are the number one undergarment problem I'm asked to solve, by actors and readers alike. If you don't actually care about this problem, you're in pretty great company! I once asked an actor if she wanted a thong, and she told me that, in fact, she loves a visible panty line. As she said to me: "I want people to know I'm wearing underwear! Can you imagine if they thought I wasn't?"

Panty lines are almost always caused by the intersection of too-tight elastic and your backside—so choosing underwear with nonbinding edges that don't cut into your flesh is obviously the best, easiest way to eradicate them. This immediately lessens the pressure of the elastic, giving you a little more breathing room and resulting in less visible skin indentations where the underwear's seams are. But the best panty line defense is really a good offense—and that means getting your underwear seams to cleverly hide themselves in the neat little shelf your butt cheeks naturally create. This is where a full-coverage garment (like the much-maligned granny panty) saves the day. When the seams and elastic follow the natural curves of your body, they disappear—and never expose themselves in the harsh light of day.

A thong is also an obvious fix for visible panty lines, but who really wants a piece of razor wire stuck up their bum all day long? If you simply *must* wear a thong with that one par-ticular pair of pants, I say maybe don't wear that pair of pants! I'm kidding, obviously—if something really requires a thong, save yourself a ton of heartache and reach for a pair of Commando brand thongs, invisible under absolutely everything and ultrasoft on your backside. I also recommend seamless boy shorts or bikini-style underwear for actors who don't want to hop on the granny-panty train. They have raw, unfinished edges that create zero bulk under clothes—making them really, truly invisible.

Mind you, these are only suggestions. The actual right pair of under-wear for you is the one that always stays firmly in place with no creep up factor. So when you finally find it, stock up! All your underwear should make you feel great, because life is hard enough already. Did you know that the average woman spends about sixteen minutes per day pulling her underwear out of her backside? Just imagine what you could get accomplished if you had those sixteen minutes back! (I actually just made that figure up, but I'd be willing to bet I'm pretty darn close to correct.)

A PANTY LINE FIX IN A PINCH

If you suddenly find your panty line is ruining an outfit (and you don't have any other options), you can try very carefully snipping the seams of your underwear at the sides (on your lower hip) to release the pressure of ultrarestrictive elastic digging into your flesh. This trick cuts visible panty lines in half instantly, but it's a true "emergency-only" fix, as said underwear are now rather unsightly. However, it will last as long as you want it to; nylon (like most synthetic fibers) doesn't tend to unravel.

YOUR GRANDMA WAS RIGHT: SLIPS RULE

In the last twenty years or so, slips somehow fell almost totally out of fashion. It's a travesty, because a wardrobe of inexpensive slips is one of the most useful things you can have in your lingerie closet. If you've ever stepped out of your house and only later realized that your dress was (whoops!) sort of see-through, well, you should've worn a slip. I've dressed reams of teenaged actors (they are actually my specialty), and every time I have a slip on the rack for one of them, she will laugh and say: "Ew, I'm not a grandma!" Then she gets into the habit of wearing one, and her life is changed for the better, forever.

In addition to keeping your dresses from being too sheer, a good slip can also help your clothes lie properly so they don't cling unflatteringly or ride up on your body. I wear a slip under almost every skirt or dress I own simply because it eliminates the dreaded "skirt stuck in butt" problem I see on the street far too often. A lot of inexpensive dresses are either unlined or have a cheap lining that bunches up and doesn't do you any favors, so the slinky anticling layer a slip provides is a god-send. If your favorite skirt or dress has a useless lining that twists and bunches uncomfortably, just cut it out with a pair of scissors and pop on a half-slip! And if you have an issue with always seeing shirt hemlines right across your bum when you tuck a shirt into a skirt, a good compression slip (think shapewear material, but in slip form) will solve the problem immediately; it gives you a firm underlayer to tuck your shirt into, hiding the seam handily. (But honestly, the only real solution to shirt hemlines that are visible through your pants or skirt is to have the shirt hemmed so the tail hits you right in the curve of your lower back, where it becomes practically invisible—head over to chapter 3 for more on brilliant alterations like this.)

I personally own and wear a ton of twelve-inch, low-rise, superstretchy microslips that are invisible underneath even the shortest of skirts. If you can't find a microslip in a pinch, just whip out a pair of scissors and convert any ancient slip you already have in your closet into a one. Nylon doesn't unravel, so you really don't even need to hem the dumb thing. A slip also helps when your overloaded handbag hikes your dress up on one side and exposes your underpants to the world. (Women in New York City who are forced to carry tote bags containing their good "going out" shoes while wearing their comfy walking shoes, I'm looking at you.) Slips keep your assets covered and cut down on wolf whistles from creepy passersby. A slip with an interesting, decorative hem can also help to lengthen a skirt that is a wee bit too short—or add some flair to a boring one. Plus—and this is the very best part of wearing a slip—when you get home at night and take off your clothes, you're already wearing part of your pajamas!

DON'T BURN YOUR BRA JUST YET...

Why do you think those groovy babes of the 1960s originally wanted to burn their bras? Yes, for equality and all, but mostly because bras are terrible torture devices! Take a seat and get comfortable, because you are about to read a bra manifesto. The whole world is obsessed with breasts—so how could any bra discussion be short, sweet, and to the point?

I once worked with a very large-busted teenage actor who told me horror story after horror story of costume designers strapping down her breasts with a compression bandage in order to hide them on camera. (She was meant to look thirteen, but Hollywood also just loves to punish beautiful, well-endowed young women who don't fit the "perfect" body mold.) I was stunned when I heard this, because her "problem" could easily have been fixed simply by putting her in the right bra.

But those three little words—"the right bra"—carry a ton of baggage with them. What is the "right" bra, anyway? The answer is as varied as the number of bodies there are in the world—because no one bra fits every person the same way. That doesn't mean that your particular body is somehow wrong; it just means you haven't found something that suits you yet. Bra shopping is the ultimate challenge for some of you, but trust me: taking the time to find a bra that fits you properly is a worthwhile endeavor. It will make every garment you have in your closet look, fit, and feel better than you could ever dream possible.

All that poor, large-busted teen actor really needed was to wear a volume-minimizing bra. They are a great way to play down what nature gave you, and also work wonders for those tops in your closet that could use a little extra help to close. A volume-minimizing bra really just shapes what was once a mountain of boob into a smoother, more manageable breast hill—using the exact same amount of dirt. No cruelty needed!

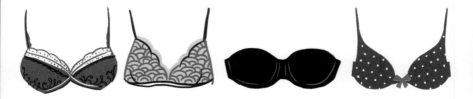

124

BRA STYLE GUIDE

If you are confused by all the styles of bra available, I'm not surprised—because there is really no standardized system of categorizing bras in the first place. Coverage, fit, and functionality vary greatly from manufacturer to manufacturer, resulting in more styles than you can shake a stick at—but I'm going to take a crack at listing all the ones you're most likely to come across.

ADHESIVE OR BACKLESS: A bra without straps that attaches to the underside of each breast and stays in place with medical-grade adhesive. Some adhesive bras incorporate silicone cups that pad and lift the breasts.

BALCONETTE: Also known as a shelf bra, this is a more revealing version of a demi-cup bra. While they offer little to no coverage, balconette bras are good for sweetheart necklines and tend to create dramatic uplift and cleavage. Balconette bras are so named because the shape of the cups is in fact a "little balcony" for each breast.

BANDEAU: A strapless band of fabric that covers the breasts. A bandeau is ultrastretchy and usually does not have built-in cups, making it a light, comfortable option for small-busted women who don't have aggressive nipples. (Larger-busted women will find a bandeau doesn't even begin to offer enough support.)

BRALETTE: An unlined, soft-cup, pullover style bra. Sometimes resembling a crop top, a bralette gives only very light support and is a comfortable alternative to traditional bras for smaller cup sizes.

BUSTIER/LONG-LINE: A highly structured undergarment that extends from bustline to high hip, distributing breast support over the entire lower torso instead of at the shoulders. This style of bra commonly closes at the back with a column of hooks and eyes and usually has flexible boning to help maintain its shape and stay wrinkle-free under clothes. Bustiers and long-line bras are perfect under special-occasion garments because they provide shaping, support, and lift without visible straps.

CONTOUR: A bra with shaped cups that mimics the natural shape of a woman's body. They often have an underwire and are usually padded or foam lined. The contour bra is the perfect choice for any woman seeking a highly sculpted silhouette, because they offer a significant amount of coverage and control.

CONVERTIBLE: A bra with detachable straps that can be reattached in a myriad of ways, depending on the needs of a particular garment. It's basically five bras in one; a convertible bra's straps can be arranged in a one shoulder, criss-cross, strapless, halter, or low-back formation.

CORSET (OVERBUST): A form-fitted support undergarment meant to slim and shape the torso, waist, and upper body to emphasize a curvy figure. A proper corset is made by a professional corsetmaker and is often fitted specifically to an individual's body. Corsets are tightened or loosened via laces at the back of the garment and often use a hook closure system at the front of the garment called a busk.

DEMI-CUP: A bra that covers half to three-quarters of the breast and extends about one inch above the nipple. This partial-cup style is designed with a slight tilt, which pushes the breasts together, creating a cleavage-enhancing shape. These bras offer less coverage than a contour bra but more than a balconette and are best for women in the A to C cup range.

FULL-CUP/FULL-FIGURE/FULL-SUPPORT: Full-cup bras completely cover the entire breast, while full-figure bras range in size from a thirty-eight-inch to a fifty-six-inch band size. Full-support bras offer maximum support, incorporating structural features designed specifically for DD+ cup sizes.

MASTECTOMY: A bra designed to hold one or two prosthetic breast inserts, which simulate the shape of an actual breast. These bras are meant for women who have had mastectomies and elected not to undergo reconstructive surgery.

NURSING: A practical bra designed to provide support for breasts that have increased in size for lactation. A nursing bra utilizes fuller cups in stretchy, nonirritating fabrics with wider shoulder straps for comfort. It aids breastfeeding via panels that can be folded down or to the side, exposing the nipple for easy access. Nursing bras do not feature underwire construction, which can restrict the flow of milk.

PADDED: A bra with shape-enhancing pads or lining designed to increase bust size. Padded bras support and "amp up" breast size, but are not intended to greatly increase cleavage.

PLUNGE: Sometimes known as a U-plunge, this is a bra designed with angled cups and a wide-open, significantly lowered center gore, allowing for increased cleavage. A plunge bra is suitable for special-occasion dresses or outfits with low necklines and is not as heavily padded as a push-up bra.

PUSH-UP: Like the original Wonderbra and Victoria's Secret Miracle Bra, this is a bra that creates the appearance of increased cleavage by using angled underwire cups and padding to push the breasts inward and upward toward the center of the chest.

RACERBACK: A bra designed with shoulder straps that form an "X" pattern at the center back for a no-show fit under tank tops or other garments that would expose traditional bra straps. A racerback bra can also provide extra support and reduce bounce for larger-busted women. (If you don't want to shell out for a proper racerback bra, flip to page 136 for my secret Hollywood-approved tips for making any bra you own a racerback for less than $5!)

SEAMLESS: A bra constructed without seamed cups. Seamless bras are a great choice for pairing with clingy knits. They are designed to be completely invisible and create a clean, uninterrupted line under clothes.

SPORTS: A bra specifically designed to offer firm support and minimize breast movement during physical activity. Usually made of stretchable, Lycra-blend fabrics, sports bras wick perspiration away from the body and reduce skin irritation due to trapped sweat.

STRAPLESS: A bra that relies on an extra-wide band and rubberized or silicone beading along the cups to support the breasts without the help of shoulder straps. Many large-busted women find that strapless bras simply will not stay up due to lack of support, so a bustier or long-line bra is a better choice for these women when faced with wearing a garment that exposes the shoulders.

T-SHIRT: A contoured-style bra designed without any front seams, hooks, or construction elements that could be seen under a T-shirt. A close cousin of the seemless bra, the T-shirt bra is almost always lined lightly with foam to help conceal the nipples.

U-BACK: Also known as a leotard-back. This is a bra that, exactly as it sounds, dips into a low "U" shape at the back closure. This type of bra features closer-set straps, which provides more support and helps prevent straps from sliding off the shoulders. A U-back bra is particularly good for full-busted or sloped-shouldered women, as straps that constantly fall down don't provide enough support.

UNDERWIRE: A bra designed with a thin, semicircular strip of rigid material (sometimes made of actual coated wire) at the bottom of each cup that helps support the breasts. Underwires are sewn directly into the bra fabric, from center gore to under the armpit.

VOLUME-MINIMIZING: A bra meant to deemphasize breasts by compressing and reshaping them. They are an intensely practical design for large-busted women because the simple readjustment of breast shape can help reduce cup spillover and alleviate pressure on the shoulders and back.

BUT DOES IT FIT?

While there is obviously no one "right" bra out there that magically suits every single body, there are definitely many bad and poorly fitted ones. The number one sign of a poorly fitted bra is its tendency to leave red marks and welts on your shoulders and ribcage. Most women are wearing their band one size too small, which is what usually causes this phenomenon. There is an entire contingent of maniacal bra fitters out there telling women that the band is supposed to be horrifyingly tight. Run, don't walk away from anyone who deems this to be okay. It's not acceptable, and a bra that digs into your flesh like a pair of satanic hawk talons is definitely not the right bra for you. For the record, only 10 percent of breast support should come from the straps—the other 90 percent should come from a properly fitted band. You should be able to easily slide two fingers under both your bra straps and your bra band. Don't just rely on too-tight straps to provide the bulk of your support! If you can fit more than two fingers under your bra band, a smaller band (that's the number in a bra size; the letter represents the size of the cup) will give the support you are currently missing out on and should also help to alleviate pain in your shoulders.

If your bra band is too large, it's likely to ride up mercilessly in the back. This concept might seem confusing until you consider the actual physics involved in how a bra provides support. It's really rather simple: to keep your breasts supported, the band of your bra must sit level (or low) on your back. When the band begins to ride up, your breasts will then drop down in front. A smaller band will sit more firmly on your rib cage and remain in place—keeping your breasts front and center where you want 'em!

A cup that is too large will sit unnaturally low on the front of the body, possibly causing your breasts to sag. If you find there is always space between the cup of your bra and your breast, try going one size down in the cup.

If you are an E cup or above, I've got some great/terrible news for you: No department or chain store bra is probably ever going to fit you. If the store in question doesn't carry your size, they are going to cram you into the closest thing they happen to have in stock and be done with it. You, my dear, are going to need to visit a real, proper, old-fashioned bra store, the kind of joint run by custom fitters who have held literally thousands of pairs of breasts in their hands. The fitter will sternly ogle your bare breasts with the detached interest of a battlefield surgeon, while her husband does crossword puzzles and mans the cash register just on the other side of the curtain. It will be a totally awkward, yet really awesome experience. (If you can't find a proper fitter in your own neighborhood, you'll need to plan ahead. This could include keeping an eye out for one in a city you may be visiting in the future, or planning a road trip with friends to a spot you found online.)

The bra your fitter recommends will most likely include a combination of letters and numbers you never dreamed possible—and will shock you with its price. You will knuckle down, buy two and treat them better than your eventual human offspring. (For all my tips on proper bra care, check out page 140). This is simply the cost of having a spectacular rack. Consider this permission to feel amazing about your boobs, because they're fabulous.

But being fitted is not the same thing as being measured. Measurements rely on a standardized method—and humans are anything but standardized. A measurement can accurately tell your band size, but your cup size really depends on your body type and shape. This is where a proper fitter can't be beat. You can measure your underbust and overbust to get an idea of bra size, but it's still just a guideline. Every brand differs, and the "size" that works so well in one brand may not fit the same in another. However, knowing how to properly measure yourself for a bra is still useful! To do it accurately, peel off your bra and start by taking a measuring tape (a soft, flexible one, that is—not one meant for measuring cabinetry!) and run it around the trunk of your body, underneath the breasts. This is your underbreast measurement—also known as your band size. Write it down; you're going to need it in a minute. (A caveat: If your underbreast measurement is an odd number, it means you should try on bras in both the size below and the size above your measurement. If your measurement is an even number, it almost always is your exact band size, but you may still need a larger or smaller size depending on body type.)

Next, lean forward at the waist so that your chest is parallel to the ground. This ensures that you'll be measuring all of your breast tissue—not just what protrudes outward while standing up. Run the tape around your torso, taking care to center it over the fullest part of your breasts. (Don't pull the tape too tightly—you want to make sure your breast tissue isn't being squished down. Also, make sure your tape measure is straight—you don't want it sliding down your back, as this will cause an inaccurate measurement. Measuring yourself in front of a mirror will help make sure the tape is staying right where you want it.) The resulting number is known as your overbust measurement, and, together with your underbust measurement, will help you figure out your likely cup size—using good old-fashioned math. To properly calculate your cup size, simply subtract your underbust measurement (also known as your band measurement, remember?) from the overbust measurement you just took. The difference between these two numbers determines your cup size. If the difference between your two measurements is less than one inch, your cup size is AA. If it's exactly one inch, you are a legit A cup. And on and on, like so:

+ Difference of two inches = B

+ Difference of three inches = C

+ Difference of four inches = D

+ Difference of five inches = DD

+ Difference of six inches = DDD (E in UK sizing)

+ Difference of seven inches = DDDD/F (F in UK sizing)

+ Difference of eight inches = G/H (FF in UK sizing)

+ Difference of nine inches = I/J (G in UK sizing)

+ Difference of ten inches = J (GG in UK sizing)

Don't be confused by the alternate UK lettering for cup sizing. I've included it here because most leading lingerie brands for sale in the United States actually use UK cup sizing above a DD. So if you see cup sizes such as a DDD or DDDD in your local lingerie shop, these are equivalent to an E and an F.

I actually consider the self-measurement method to be a far better starting point for a bra try-on session than a pushy department store salesperson. The idea that you need a clerk (who likely works on commission!) to tell you what fits and what doesn't is rather old and antiquated. I find that you're always better off to measure yourself at home and then try on a dozen bras in peace and quiet, taking your time until you land on the one that feels right to you. It's a far less awkward experience, and you aren't likely to be rushed or pressured into buying something that doesn't actually work correctly for your body just because you feel guilty that you're taking up too much of the salesperson's time.

Now that you're armed with the magic number, hop into a dressing room with a handful of bras to determine which one is best for you. While we're pretty darn sure we've arrived at the correct bra size with our clever at-home measuring, you still shouldn't take it as gospel until you've tried on bras by five different manufacturers—in five different styles. Only then will you know that your measurements told you the truth.

But let's back up for a second here. Before you can determine if a bra fits properly, you'll want to make sure you are putting it on correctly in the first place. This is not achieved by standing up straight—you actually want to lean forward the whole time to ensure that all of your breast tissue is in the bra. After removing the bra from its hanger, put your arms through the straps and lean forward slightly so that your bust falls easily into the cups. Next, fasten the bra on the largest set of hooks and eyes. While still leaning forward, grab the underwires or bottoms of each cup and give 'em a wiggle from side to side, making sure your breasts are settled comfortably and correctly into the cups. Then, slip your hand inside each cup and lift your breasts up and toward each other. At this point, you'll likely have to adjust the length of the shoulder straps. Do so by slipping each strap off your shoulders and adjusting the sliders so that the straps are short enough to stay in place without cutting into your flesh.

Next, check the band size. The correct band size is the smallest one you can comfortably wear. (This might actually be smaller than your underbust measurement, as different brands of bras have bands that stretch quite differently.) A properly fitting band should be providing the bulk of the bra's support without relying too heavily on the shoulder straps to do the work. The right-fitting bra will fit well when fastened on the loosest hook, but will be too tight if fastened on the smallest one. This is so you can comfortably tighten the band as the elastic starts to stretch and wear out. If you buy a bra that only fits on the smallest hook to start with, you won't be able to wear it once it gets to be even a little bit old!

You'll likely need to adjust your cup size when you move to a different band size. For every band size you go down, try going up by one cup size so the cups continue to have the same capacity. (And remember, a too-small cup can most definitely make the right band size seem too tight!)

I know you're getting tired of still trying on this one single bra, but there are still two steps left. Don't give up on the process now! After getting settled on the correct band size, you'll want to double-check your cup size. The correct cup size should be completely filled—with no wrinkled fabric or extra space. Any spillage means the cup size is too small—even when you're talking about low-cut or pushup bras. Check all around the cups for bulging—either at the front or at the sides under your arms. Bulging is no good and means the cups are too small.

Make sure any underwire encircles your entire breast and lies flat against your rib cage. You want the wires to sit on your ribs, not on the breast tissue. If an underwire is cutting into the sides of your breasts, you need a larger cup size. And an underwire that presses into your breastbone means you'll need to try a style with a lower center front due to the shape of your ribcage.

Finally (and most importantly!), take the time to see how the bra looks with a shirt on. You'll want to make sure that what looks great on its own also works well under your clothes. Most women find that their clothes feel and fit far better once they finally wear a bra that actually works as it should. In a properly-fitting bra, your bustline will also suddenly be at the correct proportional level—about halfway between your elbow and shoulder. If your bustline was previously riding too low due to an inadequately supportive bra, you might even find that you can suddenly wear a smaller dress size! Like I said earlier: Poor fit really is the true enemy of great style.

If you've long been plagued by armpit and back rolls, you'll be glad to know that they are often a direct result of wearing a bra that's too big in the band and too small in the cups. While bulges are sometimes caused by wearing a too-small bra, most of the time they are actually caused by a too-large bra riding up in the back. A band that sits lower on the back will remain in place—rather than migrating upward, creating bulges.

Now you know exactly how to find a bra that fits you all on your very own. See how easy that was? Who needs a snobby, sullen salesperson pressuring them into buying the wrong thing? Not you, my dear. Certainly not you.

HOW TO FRANKENSTEIN A BRA
THAT WORKS FOR YOU

Even after measuring themselves, getting properly fitted by an expert, and trying on one million and ten bras, there just may not be such a thing as the perfect bra for some women. Assuming there's a "holy grail" bra out there for all is a fairy tale. If the perfect bra doesn't exist for you, don't despair—because there are a million ways to tweak or "Frankenstein" your existing bras to perfectly suits your needs. You'll just need to use a little bit of the magic dust I keep in my bra tool kit!

HOW TO KEEP YOUR BRA STRAPS FROM FALLING DOWN

The slow bra strap slide is the most irritating wardrobe malfunction there is. Sliding bra straps have absolutely nothing to do with band size, unless you are wearing a bra that is many sizes too big. It's most likely occurring because your straps are too loose. An easy way to check your straps is to drop your shoulders and run your fingers under the straps, from the front to the highest part of your shoulder. If you can fit more than two fingers under the strap, it's too big. Your straps should never pull away from your shoulder farther than about a half inch. If they do, tighten them. Straps loosen with wear, so they need frequent adjusting.

A narrower-set strap (one that begins closer to the breast, like on a demi or balconette bra) will help address the problem somewhat, as most times, bra strap slippage is caused by wearing a style of bra that is wrong for your particular body. A woman with narrow or sloping shoulders will need to make sure a bra's straps are not set too far apart for her frame. A bra with wide-set straps can ride too close to the shoulder, resulting in the straps falling down all day long. But a bra with closer-set straps centers the bra more securely on the shoulders and back, resulting in less slippage.

An easy no-sew option to keep bra straps from sliding all over the place is to use a set of old-school, pin-in lingerie strap keepers. They are the original solution to bra strap slippage, used by broads like Joan Crawford since the dawn of modern fashion. Essentially a thin piece of ribbon with a snap sewn on each end, you pin them into your garment at the shoulder (taking care to only allow the pin to grab the innermost layer of fabric so that it doesn't show) and then snap them around your bra straps—and just like that, your straps stop sliding southward. They are about two bucks at any sewing or notions joint. (You can also use them to keep your straps in place with an off the shoulder or boat neck–style shirt.) Some "better" or vintage garments have these lingerie straps already sewn in, and I'll bet a bunch of you reading this right now thought those tiny ribbons with snaps were just meant to keep the clothes on the hanger while in the store. If you're feeling fancy, you can have a tailor stitch a set of these "bra keepers" into your favorite garments for about $7 a pair.

Making your bra a halter is another surefire way to keep your straps in place. I use a simple plastic racerback clip—available at almost any store that has a decent lingerie department—but you can also use a large safety pin to make any bra into a halter in a pinch. (Just make sure to let your bra straps down a little longer before you halter up.) As a bonus, if you happen to have wide-spaced breasts, making your bra a halter will pull them together, resulting in a more supportive fit.

Another cheap, easy solution to slipping bra straps is to slap a piece of Topstick tape onto your bra straps at the shoulders and then adhere them to your shirt. They will stay put all day long until you don't want them to anymore, then peel off with ease. If you are a babe who has to wear a bra with exactly everything, this is the tip of a lifetime for you. It's also why you never see an actor's bra straps showing on TV! Topstick is an integral part of my costume kit, and it's available at almost any sewing or wardrobe supply store (see page 78 for more).

HOW TO STOP BRA STRAPS FROM DIGGING INTO YOUR FLESH

One word: Ouch. Bra straps dig into your tender shoulder flesh for many reasons. Sometimes, it's simply breast size—boobs are really heavy! But other times, it's caused by the bra—or the strap itself. If you suffer from digging straps, make sure you are wearing a bra with flat-style strap, not a rounded string style. Also make sure that your straps are wide enough for your cup size. The bigger the cup, the wider the strap should be. A wider strap provides a firmer base of support, so the weight of each breast is then spread evenly across your shoulder—not focused on one thin pressure point as with a thin, rounded strap. You can also look for bras with padded straps or invest in an inexpensive pair of silicone strap cushions, available at specialty bra shops or from your old pal, the Internet.

A too-soft bra (like a flimsy silk bra) can be prone to excessive stretchiness, allowing your straps to dig fiercely into your shoulders. Make sure the bra you choose is made from a rigid enough material, such as a sturdy compression fabric—as the less give in the band and cups, the less work the straps have to do. You don't want it to be stiff or tight—just sturdy and supportive.

HOW TO MAKE A BRA FIT USING AN EXTENDER

People get all hung up on bra extenders, those rectangular pieces of material that latch onto both ends of your bra, giving you extra room by acting as a sort of patch. People like to claim that if you're fitted correctly, you shouldn't ever have to use one—and that an extender means you're wearing the wrong bra. I'll never understand the bellyaching about their very existence, because the truth is, some people just need them! For example, women with broader backs and smaller cups have a notoriously hard time finding bras—so if your band size is large and your cup size is small, you're kind of out of luck. But in this case, buying a bra that fits well in the cup but is two inches too small in the band and using an extender isn't a failure—it's a brilliant (and necessary) life hack. So use one, have a bra that fits, and be foxy.

HOW TO FIGHT BACK BULGE

A properly fitting bra (one where the band sits low on your back, not way up near your shoulder blades, remember?) should help prevent your skin from pouring out over said bra. I call this phenomenon "overhang," but you may know it as "back fat." It's just a sad fact of life—as I've seen it on skinny and plus-sized actors alike. It could mean your bra is too tight—but since a bra's band is what needs to provide the bulk of breast support, overhang could still be a problem, even if you go up a size. Some people just have looser skin than others! If skin overhang is your cross to bear in life, look for a bra with two, not three hooks and higher sides to keep everything tucked in. This creates a larger area of coverage and support—which helps distribute pressure, resulting in less bulging.

A softer, stretchier bra can sometimes help to alleviate overhang, while a more rigid bra has the tendency to accentuate it. I realize this sounds like the exact opposite of what I just recommended for straps that dig into your shoulders, but different things work for different folks—and half of finding what works for you is trial and error.

HOW TO WEAR BACKLESS STUFF WITH A BRA

Wearing a bra with a backless shirt and keeping it out of sight is a pointless battle—unless you use a low-back bra converter. This handy piece of elastic hooks onto both sides of your existing bra clasp and wraps around the front of your lower stomach, pulling the band down in back while still offering maximum support in front.

If you can sew on a button, you can make your own bra extender with a piece of elastic and some hooks you've cannibalized from an ancient, stretched out bra. Heck, you could really just safety pin those hook ends onto the elastic and be done with it.

If your garment is both backless and strapless, you should try wearing a long-line bra. Some folks consider it to be a dated style, but a long-line bra dips low in the back and derives its support from a corset-like bodice—which has the added benefit of smoothing lumps and looking sleek under clothes. Once you get used to wearing it, you'll wonder how you ever lived without one in heavy rotation. If you are large busted, you may have thought that a strapless bra was forever outside the realm of possibility for you due to the utter lack of support and constant slippage. A long-line bra stays up due to the built-in support of the bodice—which basically stabilizes your boobs on a handy little shelf. It's a great alternative to the classic strapless bra that heads southward with the slightest hint of any motion—such as daring to lift your arms over your head at a party.

HOW TO GO WITHOUT A BRA

I love going braless—but am also quite interested in keeping my nipples under wraps whenever I venture outside. Self-adhesive silicone nipple covers (available at better lingerie and department stores for about $10) are perfection for those who can go without a bra and just need a touch of modesty. But they also work just as well for women who practically have to sleep in their bras—because sometimes even the best bra can't stop nipples that insist on perking up whenever they please. A well-made pair of nipple covers should be washable and reuseable up to thirty times with careful use.

HAND WASHING YOUR BRAS AND UNDIES

You most likely already knew this, but you should be hand washing your better bras and underwear, period. And washing your bras in the shower while bathing (you'd be surprised at the emails I get!) isn't going to cut it—unless you're using laundry-grade soap, which is terrible for your skin. Take the time to hand wash your bras once every two weeks by soaking them in the bathroom sink in warm water with a capful of gentle laundry soap or baby shampoo for about ten minutes, then rinsing well. Take care not to wring, twist, or press your bras, which can cause them to lose their shape. When you think you're done rinsing, rinse once more for good measure—excess soap attracts dirt and makes your bras wear out faster. Once you're done, lay your clean, wet bra cups up on a dry towel until it is no longer dripping wet, then finish air-drying by hanging it from both straps on a hanger in an area where air can move through it freely. Make sure your bras are properly reshaped before you set them aside to dry—if the cups get dented while being washed, take your fingers and gently smooth them out so they look like cups again.

If you must toss your bras in the washer due to lack of time or extreme laziness, invest in a plastic bra-washing ball or structured wash bag. Hook all hooks and clasp all clasps before washing to avoid excess twisting and snagging. And never put your bras in the dryer—most bras are made of synthetic materials and can't withstand the heat. (It'll also damage the wire.) But even if you toss your bras in the washer and dryer like a wild woman, I still love you. And your boobs are still spectacular.

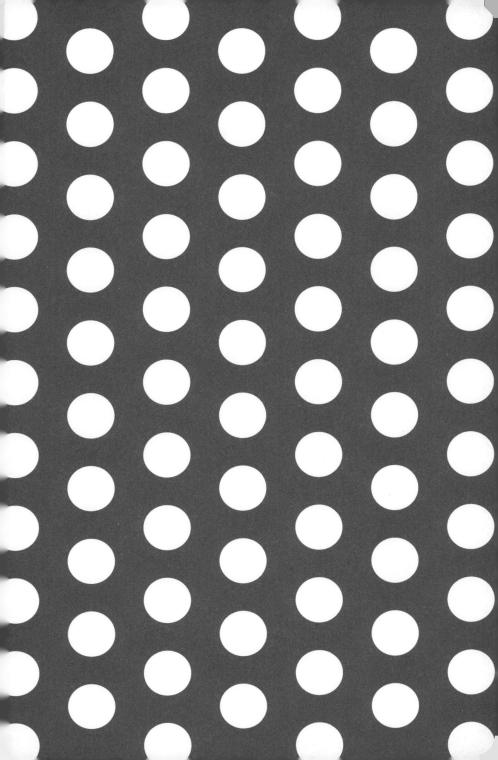

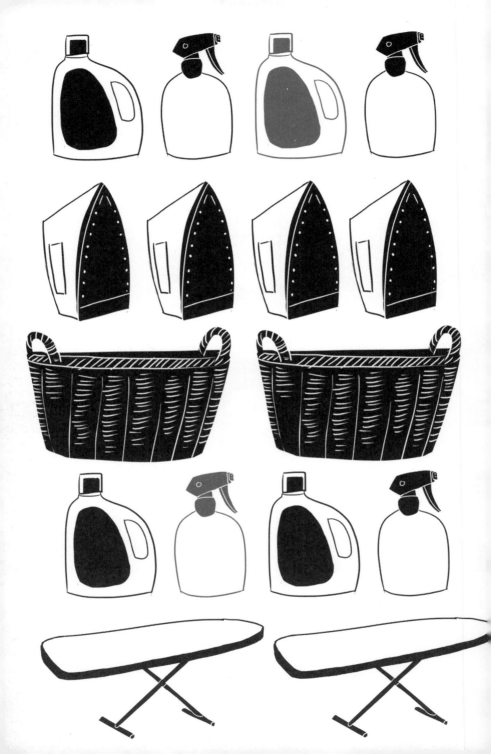

CHAPTER 10

LAUNDRY:
you're doing it wrong

Doing laundry seems so easy, right? Open washer, stuff in clothes, run on any random cycle, toss in dryer on hottest heat, heap the results in a laundry basket, and you're done. But if that's even close to your current laundry shtick, guess what? You're totally doing it wrong. A little extra time and effort can go a very long way toward extending the life of your clothes. You could have the fantasy closet of your wildest dreams, stuffed to the gills with fancy frocks—but every bit of it would be pointless if you don't know how to take care of it.

It's sad, but the art of laundry has somehow completely fallen out of fashion in recent years. It used to be that clothes were either dreadfully expensive, or you had to make them yourself. As a result, people didn't have a ton of them, so knowing how to wash and care for them properly was super important. The epic rise of fast fashion has made clothes practically throwaway, so many of us don't really care if something gets ruined in the wash—but some of your favorite pieces may also happen to be things you actually didn't pay very much for, so I'm sure you'd like to maintain and wear them for years to come. You also likely own a few pieces of more expensive clothing that you don't want ruined. The art of laundry is important—and was taught to me at a young age by both of my grandmothers, working in tandem to turn me into the lean, mean, laundry machine I am today. I'm actually a laundry enthusiast! So allow me to take you on a journey—deep into the wild, wonderful world of proper laundry practices. I promise you, I'm an excellent tour guide.

GET THE MOST OUT OF YOUR WASHING MACHINE

Before you even begin to do laundry, you'll want to take a minute to familiarize yourself with the machines you'll be using—and to make sure you're using the right type of laundry soap for your particular machine. If your washer is a high-efficiency model, always use detergent that is marked "HE" specifically for such washers. While it may seem unnecessary, these washers actually use far less water than traditional machines—and therefore need a detergent that is low-sudsing. Using a non-HE laundry detergent in an HE machine can result in an overwhelming amount of suds that leaves a sticky film on your clothes.

If you are washing a load of black or very dark clothing, consider investing in a detergent made specifically for dark clothing. It will pay off in the long run; these detergents help cut down on fading immensely. I love Woolite's "Darks" laundry detergent to keep all my fancy jeans and vintage black concert T-shirts looking new and crisp.

YOU HAVE TO START SOMEWHERE, SO WHY NOT SORT PROPERLY?

I love sorting laundry, because proper sorting will cause your clothes to live longer, happier lives. It's really your best defense against ruined clothes! There are six distinct categories into which you should be separating your laundry. (I swear, it's not as hard as it sounds.) Stay with me, because the end results are well worth it:

WHITES OR LIGHTS: A load of lights and whites means that only very pale-colored or white T-shirts, cotton undies, pajamas, and the like go together—basically anything that is light enough to not bleed onto other garments. (I consider pale yellow to be the darkest color you can safely put in a load of lights.) Wash lights in warm water for maximum grime removal, as T-shirts and undies tend to get the most foul of all your laundry.

BRIGHTS: In laundry, as in life, red means danger. Red clothing is laundry enemy number one, as it is notorious for turning an entire load of whites pale pink. You can wash reds, bright oranges, hot pinks, and deep purples together once you are completely sure they are colorfast. For extra insurance, you can toss a color catching sheet (like the Shout Color Catcher sheet, available in the laundry soap aisle of the drugstore) in with your bright loads to help trap any excess dye that could deposit itself on other garments. I always test colorfastness by spraying the garment with water in a discreet spot and then blotting with a paper towel to see if any dye transfers. If you like, you can go a step further and swish the item around in a sink of warm water to see if it releases any color. This may seem like an annoying extra step, but you will thank me profusely later when you preemptively save your favorite blouse. I wash brights in cold water only, which helps cut down on color fade.

DARKS: Your darks load should include stuff like jeans, sweatshirts, and gym clothes—basically any garment that can stand up to the dye in a pair of blue jeans. But a warning: If your jeans are brand new, wash them alone until they finish their dye purge. (It will be obvious that they are done purging once your thighs stop turning blue after wearing them, which should be after about five washes.) I wash my really good jeans in cold water as infrequently as possible and always inside out to help prevent fading, making sure to take them out of the dryer while they are slightly damp to prevent scorching and shrinking. I wash darks in cold or warm water, depending on the grime level. Whoever said heat sets a stain was only half right: once you *dry* a stain with heat, it's yours for life—but warm water is the ticket if you've got clothes that are extra, extra dirty.

GENTLE OR COLD: I keep anything delicate, silky, linen, or vintage out of the regular wash. This includes fancy underwear, bras, slips, and stuff that just seems like it would get beat up by hot water and a super-aggressive spin cycle. Even cheap polyester dresses can benefit from the extra care the gentle cycle and cold water gives. Cold water puts less stress on the fibers—and when they take less of a beating, they don't pill or fray quite as easily. Wash your delicates in a load by themselves with your washer set to gentle, using mesh laundry bags so the delicates don't get hammered to death by the spin cycle. A mesh bag is also a good way to make sure your socks don't get lost in the wash, if you are a person who values such a thing. With the exception of said socks, make sure to never put anything you deem mesh bag or gentle cycle–worthy in the dryer. It's all drip dry, all the time, baby.

HOUSEHOLD LINENS: If you've ever accidentally washed a bath towel with some of your clothes, you already know that they produce a special kind of lint that attaches itself to your wardrobe forever, like lice on a first grader. For that reason alone, household linens should be washed by themselves. But the other reason is because *ewww, grime, food particles, body fluids, yuck*! Wash towels, sheets, and kitchen rags in the hottest water possible to help fight grime.

OTHERS: There are always random items in my wardrobe that are half dark and half white or have some other weird characteristic that makes me scratch my head as to how to sort them. Shirts that have a white body with dark sleeves always stress me out in particular. I wash them by themselves in a mini-load with cold water the first few times to see how they behave, then sort accordingly from that point on.

HOW TO GET YOUR CLOTHES REALLY, REALLY CLEAN

Hot water kills bacteria and deodorizes naturally. If everything you are washing is pure white, add a quarter-cup of chlorine bleach to really amp up the clean. But don't overdo it; too much bleach turns everything yellow and can eat right through the fibers. If you find that your smelly gym clothes don't get fully clean with detergent alone, add either a cup of baking soda at the start of the wash as a detergent booster or a cup of white vinegar in the rinse cycle to help neutralize odor. If your clothes start to look dingy, there's a huge chance they are suffering from detergent buildup. Make sure not to over use soap—and consider using your machine's extra rinse cycle if you still see bubbles or white residue after washing.

YOUR FINAL LAUNDRY SECURITY CHECKPOINT

Check everything you're about to wash and dry for stains and pretreat them accordingly. (Not sure how to treat a particular stain? Check out my actor-tested, costume-designer approved stain-removal tricks on page 157–64.) Like I said before, once you heat-dry a stain, it's never leaving your side—so make sure it is really gone before tossing your clothes into the washer and dryer. If your stains are of the terrible yellow underarm variety, I'm sad to say that all hope is almost certainly lost. You can try blasting them beyond recognition with a homemade paste of dishwashing liquid, hydrogen peroxide, and baking soda, scrubbing the affected area with an old toothbrush. It sometimes works, but only on plain white, 100 percent cotton garments.

I know an actor who sprays the armpits of his white T-shirts with a very light coating of adhesive spray (like you'd use to mount photos onto posterboard for a science project, available at any art supply store) and then runs a warm iron over the area to "set" it before he wears them each time to keep the underarms free of yellowed pit stains. I thought this idea was crazy until he further explained that the glue acts to "seal up" the spaces in between the T-shirt's threads, preventing dirt, sweat, and grime from really settling in the underarm area. I finally tried it myself, and—holy laundry tip, Batman!—it really works. Just take care not to spray too much adhesive (or use too high of an iron setting) to avoid scorching. But keep in mind that this solution is meant to be preventative. Sadly, it can do nothing for you once underarm stains are already in residence.

As you sort, make sure to check all pockets for money, tissues, gum, pens, lipstick, and other random objects that could foul up your clothes. By the time you see an uncapped lipstick floating by itself in the middle of the wash cycle, it's too late. Be sure to button all buttons, zip all zippers, and snap all snaps. This helps lessen fastener breakage and stops garments from getting incredibly twisted in the wash.

START YOUR WASHERS!
You are finally ready to do some laundry. Can you believe it? But before you do, determine what the proper load size is for your washer. Overloading means that not enough water and soap can work their way into your garments, preventing your clothes from getting really clean. Everything should be packed in the washer loosely, not tightly, like a

bowl of chunky chicken soup. A regular-capacity washer holds one bed sheet, four pillowcases, two or three shirts, and about six pairs of underwear (not that you should be washing all those things together! It's just to give you a visual.) A loosely packed laundry basket is about the right amount.

BUT WAIT—WE'RE NOT FINISHED YET!

You've likely just successfully done your laundry exactly right. But you're not quite finished—because you still have to get it dry somehow. Before you toss your clothes in the dryer, take the time to unroll any wadded up hems, sleeves, or pant legs. Giving everything a good snap and shake out before you dry cuts wrinkles in half. Try not to overload or underload your dryer—if you have too few clothes in the load, the dryer can't properly tumble, lengthening your drying time (and costing you more money). If your dryer is too full, air won't be able to circulate evenly and you'll pull still-damp, wrinkled items out of the dryer even after an hour of tumbling. As with your washer load, a normal-sized laundry basket that is packed like a bowl of chunky chicken soup is the exact right amount for optimal drying action.

Don't mix your loads in the dryer—like with like ensures that nothing ever gets overdried. I like to take stuff out of the dryer while it's just this side of damp—any longer and things start shrinking quite rapidly. Becoming religious about hanging everything up while still slightly damp and allowing it to finish drying by air extends the life of your clothes exponentially. (It's also a really good way to save quarters at the laundromat!) Your clothes (even your jeans) should always be dried on low or medium heat only—high heat is too hot and is strictly reserved for towels and sheets. Fragile fabrics such as spandex and elastic do best on a short, "cool air only" cycle. When you take your items out of the dryer, be sure to give them a vigorous shake out and line up all seams before folding. This ensures that no "secret wrinkles" get etched into your garments (you know, the kind that only another washing could possibly remove).

Don't forget to check the lint trap every time you dry a load—both inside the machine and at the back where the exhaust is. Clogged lint screens impact the efficiency of your dryer and can even start fires. I only use dryer sheets for clothes that are very prone to static as they can add a coating to bath towels that tends to render them a little less absorbent.

OH, ONE MORE THING...

Even if you've dutifully taken everything out of the dryer ASAP, snapped the wrinkles out, and straightened the seams like a good little laundry bunny, chances are you'll still have a handful of items that need some help. While I'm a pretty big proponent of steaming over ironing (which I waxed poetic about way back in chapter 6), having a few ironing smarts in your back pocket is a necessary life skill—because sometimes, you may only have access to a good old-fashioned iron. But if you've ever ruined a garment with a too-hot or dirty iron, you're probably a little apprehensive about the process. The number one thing you can do to avoid damage to your clothes is to always to start ironing on one setting cooler than what you think your garment needs. You can always crank up the heat if need be, but you can't undo the iron-plate shaped scorch mark that comes from pressing a silky garment with an iron set to stun. If your iron has a buildup of brown, burned-on residue, don't attempt to use it until you've gotten it clean. There are a handful of home remedies for scorched iron gunk, but I've never had any of them work even a little bit. It's commercial iron cleaner or bust, as far as I'm concerned.

To protect your clothes, iron garments inside out as often as you can. Use short, even strokes, going with the grain of the fabric and keeping the iron moving at all times. A resting iron is an iron that is damaging your clothes. A slightly moist pressing cloth (like a thin kitchen towel or cotton dinner napkin) will help press out stubborn wrinkles while protecting delicate fabrics from burning and scorching. I steam almost everything I can, but certain items (such as those with intricate folds or pleats) just need a good ironing.

For shirts, start by ironing the underside of the collar, followed by the sleeves and back. Finish off your shirt pressing by running the iron over the the shirt's front. When ironing pleated items, start at the bottom of each fold and work up toward the top of the garment. (Pressing pleated items at home is a small challenge, but it's also a huge part of skipping out on hefty dry-cleaning bills—so you owe it to yourself to at least try!) To properly iron a pair of pants, start with the inside pockets, waistband, backside, and front, working down to the crotch before moving on down the legs. Be sure to hang them by their cuffs on a clip hanger to maintain all your difficult ironing work!

LASTLY, SHOW YOUR MACHINES SOME LOVE

You may not realize it, but your washer needs a little TLC every so often. Make sure to run it empty with a cup or two of white vinegar every few months to keep things clean. (A cup of antiseptic mouthwash works too!) After running your vinegar or mouthwash load, wipe down the inside of the machine, lid, and seals with a wet cloth. Also, does your washing machine stink? Mine, too! High-efficiency and front-loading machines are way more likely to collect mold and mildew than regular old top loaders because they have air and watertight seals. Cleaning your machine regularly (including scrubbing the rubber seal on the door) with a mixture of hot water, bleach, and vinegar will help the problem, but the real solution is far easier—just leave the door open for about twenty minutes so the drum can dry out between washings. (But proceed with caution if you have kids or pets.) You can also sprinkle a little baking soda in the drum after every wash to help absorb odors.

If your washer is leaving rust spots on your clothes, the enamel has most likely chipped off somewhere inside. A little sanding and painting with a bit of rustproof paint is a way easier repair than it sounds, I promise. Treat your machines well—and they will treat your clothes like royalty. It's never too late to start down the road to doing your laundry right, especially now that you are a certified laundry artiste just like me! Your wardrobe will thank you for it.

IS DRY-CLEANING REALLY NECESSARY?

You may be wondering what the hell dry-cleaning even is—I myself thought it was just sheer wizardry until I went on a field trip to the plant that handles my show costumes. As I was walking around learning all about the process, a shocking thought entered my mind: "What if dry-cleaning isn't actually necessary?" I didn't dare pose the question to my lovely dry cleaner while I was his guest, but I couldn't stop wondering if the entire dry-cleaning industry was really just sort of a scam, meant to scare us into paying someone else to take care of our clothes. What if there was a way to cut out all the time and expense associated with dragging your clothes back and forth across town just to get them clean?

You won't find many dry cleaners who will admit it, but the truth is that dry-cleaning sort of isn't necessary at all. In most cases, it's simply a luxury. There is almost nothing marked "Dry-Clean Only" that you can't safely wash yourself at home—for um, practically free. The only reason my dry cleaner was finally willing to admit that my theory was correct is because he does not serve the general public—he strictly does dry-cleaning for television and film shoots, so if you skip the dry cleaner, it doesn't hurt his business one bit. When shooting wraps at midnight and we have to be back on set bright and early at 7:00 a.m., there's no way we are going to stay up and hand wash our actors' clothes to be ready the next morning. We simply call the dry cleaner, who picks everything up from us right on stage, no matter what the hour, and returns it to us bright and early the next morning before we've even reported to work. We could carefully hand wash everything and have it look just as good as when it came from the dry cleaner, but we obviously don't have the time. However, you do, so take heed! Your clothes (and your wallet) will thank you for it, since dry-cleaning isn't actually all that good for clothes anyway. Over time, the chemicals used can cause fabric to break down and shrink irreparably.

Dry-cleaning came about in the mid-nineteenth century when a dye-shop owner noticed that his tablecloth was markedly cleaner in the spot where he'd spilled some kerosene, a known solvent. Voila! Modern dry-cleaning was born. But is dry-cleaning really "dry"? And how can anything get clean when it doesn't actually get wet? It turns out that professional dry-cleaning gets your clothes clean almost the same way you do at home—except that your garments are "washed" using fluid solvents instead of old-fashioned soap and water to dissolve dirt and grime. Everything gets loaded into a giant washing machine and bathed in a chemical solution that breaks down stains, soils, and grease while still retaining the fabric's shape and luster. Your local dry cleaner also has an iron as big as a dining room table, so it's no sweat for them to press six dozen shirts in the time it takes you to get one garment looking halfway presentable.

SO WHEN IS "DRY-CLEAN ONLY" NOT REALLY "DRY-CLEAN ONLY"?

Nine times out of ten, it's true that dry-cleaning is actually not necessary. But there *are* a handful of things that should never, ever be put in the washing machine or even washed by hand, no matter how broke you happen to be. I've compiled a glossary of fabric types and specific care instructions for you to refer to on page 225, but you should also read the care label in each garment carefully to determine what really, really needs to hit the dry cleaners—and what you can actually wash at home using a little TLC. And take heed: Wool suits with lining, anything made of leather, suede, fur, feathers, acetate or taffeta pieces (a.k.a. bridesmaid's dress material), and silk velvet are all things you should take directly to a professional dry cleaner—do not pass go and do not collect $200! Here's why:

+ Suit lining is usually made of acetate, which has a tendency to shrink mercilessly upon contact with water.

+ Most wool suits also have some sort of glue at the front of the jacket to attach the exterior fabric to the interior canvas and help it keep its shape. Water is the enemy of glue, so always send your wool suits out for professional dry-cleaning.

+ Leather, suede, fur, and feathers also need special care—they are natural materials that lost their water-resistant properties once they were no longer attached to the animal they came from. (A side note: There are some instances where you can actually wash suede—keep an eye out for hides that have been treated with special enzymes and that are labeled "washable suede." However, never put suede—washable or otherwise—into the dryer.)

+ Due to its heavy nap, silk velvet can be impossible to reshape once it's gotten wet.

But beyond those few specific items, almost any 100 percent natural fiber (including silk, linen, chiffon, and cashmere), in addition to lightly beaded or sequined items and practically all synthetics (such as nylon, polyester, and acrylic), can safely be washed at home—*as long as you are careful*. Yes, even knitted wool sweaters! And yes, I said sequins—hand washing sequined and beaded pieces is actually far better for them, as dry-cleaning fluid can sometimes melt the trim right off a garment. (Just make sure the trim is stitched on, not glued, before attempting hand washing.) When things are labeled "Dry-Clean Only," it's usually just the manufacturers covering their butts in case something goes wrong with your home hand washing attempts.

One caveat: Certain very brightly colored, patterned silks have a tendency to bleed mercilessly, marring the print, so I'd suggest always sending them to the dry cleaner. The same goes for pieces with ultracomplicated construction such as pleats or origami-like folds, and anything lined. Linings in particular have a terrible tendency to shrink and twist when washed, so I never take a chance.

TO SKIP THE DRY CLEANER, YOU'D BETTER LEARN HOW TO HAND WASH

If, after careful review, the garment seems like it can be safely hand washed, give it a dunk in a sink or bucket full of slightly warm water and a capful of gentle detergent (or good old-fashioned baby shampoo). If you are washing a cashmere or wool sweater, add a small squirt of hair conditioner or fabric softener to the water as well—it helps keep the fibers from drying out. (A few drops of lavender oil is a good idea, too—it naturally repels moths and weevils, those twin devils that love to eat wool and cashmere.) Cold water is also good for hand washing, but isn't quite as effective at removing dirt and odors.

It takes a good five minutes of constant movement in the wash bath to really get an item clean. Yes, that means you'll have to stand there the whole time and carefully swish your dirty garment around in a sink full of water. Don't freak out if you see some dye bleed into the water—if it's a solid color garment, I promise you won't notice any color loss once you're finished. Take great care not to rub the garment against itself—there's no need to act like a pioneer woman beating your clothes against a rock. Excess friction is exactly what causes fabrics to weaken, stretch, and pill. To rinse, let the dirty water drain completely and then refill the sink as many times as it takes until the water stays clean. As tempting as it is to squeeze the garment under running water, avoid doing so! It can easily damage delicate fibers. The goal is to avoid disturbing them as much as possible.

After rinsing, don't wring or twist your item—lay it flat on a clean, dry towel and roll it up into a burrito to squeeze all the water out of it while still retaining its shape. Repeat the burrito process until the item is nearly dry, then lay it flat to dry on another towel (taking care to coax the item back into shape with your fingers if needed), making sure air can freely circulate around it. Never, ever put an item you've just spent all that time hand washing into the dryer—it is the death of delicate fabrics! You'd be better off letting a pack of jackals shred your hand-washables to pieces; it would accomplish the same thing but be far more entertaining.

If a wool sweater accidentally finds its way into the dryer and is now shrunken to the point where it would only fit a doll, you can try submerging it in a solution of one gallon cool water to one-half cup of hair conditioner for about a half hour, then laying it flat (without rinsing) and gently working the fibers apart in an outward motion. It usually works, because what causes the wool to shrink in the first place is water getting in between the fibers and snarling them—and hair conditioner helps to "untangle" them, just like it does for ratty, knotted hair.

Once your garments have air dried, the real work begins. Pressing is a job in and of itself—it's really the main thing you're paying the dry cleaner for! (Having someone else press your clothes is my personal definition of luxury.) As soon as your item is about 98 percent dry, get to work carefully pressing the inside-out garment back into shape with a medium-warm iron. (And be sure to use an old T-shirt or handkerchief as a pressing cloth between the iron plates and the garment.) Or, you could do like wardrobe girls do and gently coax your clean garment back into shape using the power of steam like we talked about back on page 87.

You're probably reading this thinking "Geez, this hand washing sure sounds like a lot of work!" Well, yes, it is, but just think of all the money you'll manage to save on dry-cleaning bills. I'd rather spend my money on lipsticks and cocktails any day. Learning how to carefully hand wash things you previously thought were "dry-clean only" also allows you to splurge on pieces you previously wouldn't have, because now you know how to safely get them clean at home. Professional dry-cleaning is an amazing modern marvel, but every single solvent-laden cleaning lessens the life of your garments—so if you can manage to do it less often, you're extending the amount of time that you'll be able to enjoy your clothes.

In between hand washings and dry-cleanings, you can easily "freshen up" your special-care garments with an at-home dry-cleaning system, available at your local grocery store for about $15. It isn't meant to replace professional dry-cleaning, but it's great for getting odors out and buying you a few extra wearings between washings or professional cleanings. Suit jackets and pants come out beautifully using an at-home dry-cleaning process, but I'd absolutely *never* use an at-home system on any leather, feathered, fur, or beaded item.

The biggest hurdle in determining if you can safely wash something on your own is knowing what you're working with in the first place. If you've ever looked at the fabric description of a garment online or in a store and wondered what the heck it meant, you are not alone. Even I'm left scratching my head sometimes. There are just too many types of fabrics for one person to keep straight! The simple Fabric Glossary on page 225 will help shed a little light on how to care for whatever you've got—no matter what it happens to be made of.

STAINS: OR, SPIT REMOVES BLOOD LIKE WHOA

I learned how to get stains out of clothes like a pro on one of my very first costume jobs. I was a wardrobe assistant on a made-for-TV movie (which was so incredibly terrible, it never actually made it to your particular television) that featured a chorus line of male dancers wearing Santa Claus thongs. (And I'm not talking about the shoe version of thongs, either.) I dutifully sent those Santa thongs out to be laundered daily, but every so often, they'd come back . . . well, not entirely clean. And when there's a terrible, gross, or gruesome task to be done in the wardrobe department, it falls to the lowest person on the totem pole—and on this particular job, that was me. (Oh, and in case you're wondering, I used a combination of rubber gloves, dish soap, and elbow grease to get those thongs totally clean.)

Stains on clothes have likely plagued the human race since the dawn of time. I'm sure the first recorded stain in history was experienced by a caveperson who was cursing as meat juice or blood ran down his or her animal skin garment. Assuming this caveperson cared about such problems, they probably unknowingly yet instinctively applied the absolute perfect remedy to their bloody stain problem: saliva. Spit really is the best cure for bloodstains of any sort—if you can stomach it. The "old wives'" tale is that it needs to be your own spit to remove your own blood due to some antibodies nonsense, but the truth is that, really, anybody's saliva will be effective at removing bloodstains.

Saliva works on blood because they are both organic materials. The idea that it needs to be your own saliva probably arose out of your own personal mouth usually being the most convenient mouth available when blood gets shed. I get blood on actors' clothes all the time, because I am an aggressive pinner who refuses to use a thimble. I've never, ever stabbed an actor with a pin unless it was completely intentional, but I've stabbed myself somewhere in the neighborhood of one thousand times—and I almost always draw blood. I like to wait until the garment is off the actor's body before I start licking it, but time really is of the essence when you've got a stain. A fresh one is far easier to remove than one that's even just a few hours old.

Building on the knowledge that spit removes blood, it makes sense that an enzyme-based stain remover is indeed your best bet for large-scale blood removal (I won't ask), grass, dirt, food, urine, coffee, or other organic stains—because organic stains are themselves enzyme-based stains. If you've ever taken a chemistry class, you already know the golden rule of solvents: like removes like. Enzyme-based cleaners such as Zout Triple Enzyme Formula (beware of OxiClean, which can inadvertently lighten delicate fabrics) contain complex molecules made by living organisms that actually work to digest their fellow organic, protein-based stains—much like the digestive juices in your stomach break down food to aid in digestion! But this doesn't mean you should start your stain removal process with a commercially available product—those should be a matter of last resort. Oftentimes, the simplest solution is also the best—and that would be plain old water.

Ice-cold water is all you need to remove most stains—it's a universal solvent. If a material (such as denim, cotton, polyester or pure silk) can take it, flushing or gently dabbing the stain with water is often all you'll need to do to release it, especially if it's fresh. If the stain is oily or greasy, sprinkle a little talc or baby powder on it to soak up as much matter as possible before moving on to flushing it with water. Let the powder sit for a few minutes, then gently blow it off the surface to avoid grinding in the stain. Rinse or flush with cold water immediately.

For fragile or delicate fabrics like chiffon or silk, use distilled water instead—the lack of minerals helps to avoid leaving a water "ring" or wet spot on your garment. Never rub at a stain, no matter how tempting it may be. Blotting and dabbing the stain with a clean white cloth are your best bets. (We keep a pack of cloth baby diapers on set for this exact purpose!) If plain water doesn't do the trick, move on to adding a few drops of a detergent made for delicate fabrics mixed with a few drops of 3 percent hydrogen peroxide to the stain, applying the mixture carefully with a cotton swab. The marriage of hydrogen peroxide and gentle laundry detergent is exceedingly good at removing stains because the peroxide acts as an oxidizer, which leeches out the color compounds and pigments that are present in practically every stain one could acquire!

Some pigments are harder to remove than others with just plain water because they aren't water soluble in the first place—but the soap molecules in detergent latch themselves onto those pigment stains while the peroxide goes to work on the color compounds, creating a gentle chemical reaction that blasts stains out of the park without damaging your garment. Allow your peroxide and detergent mixture to sit on the stain for fifteen minutes (less on delicate fabrics like chiffon), and then rinse thoroughly with ice-cold water if the fabric can take it—otherwise blot repeatedly with cold water (or distilled water) and a clean cloth to neutralize the peroxide.

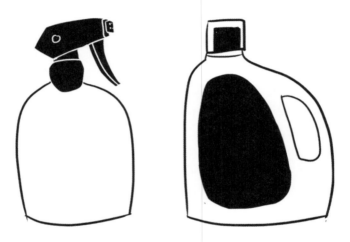

Commercial stain removers and home remedies are meant to be employed only after both plain water and the hydrogen peroxide-plus-detergent trick has failed. In stain removal, as in life, don't bring out the big guns until you really need to. But certain stains just call for a little bit more firepower to be added to the mix. And that means building your own personal stain-fighting kit, identical to the one I use on set:

BUILD YOUR OWN STAIN KIT

—

+ 3 PERCENT HYDROGEN PEROXIDE

+ BABY POWDER

+ BLUNT KITCHEN KNIFE

+ CLEAN DISH SPONGES

+ CLEAN WHITE CLOTHS

+ CLEAN WHITE TOWELS

+ DISTILLED WATER

+ ENZYME-BASED STAIN REMOVER (LIKE ZOUT TRIPLE ENZYME FORMULA)

+ GLASS EYEDROPPER

+ LIQUID DISHWASHING DETERGENT

+ LIQUID LAUNDRY DETERGENT

+ PAPER GROCERY BAGS

+ PAPER TOWELS

+ PROFESSIONAL DRY-CLEANING FLUID OR AT-HOME DRY-CLEANING KIT

+ RUBBER GLOVES

+ RUBBING ALCOHOL

+ WATERLESS MECHANIC'S SOAP (LIKE MECHANIC'S FRIEND)

+ WHITE VINEGAR

Armed with these simple tools, you can perform the exact same stain-removing magic tricks I do on my actors' clothes daily. While some of them may have you scratching your head as to their purpose, I swear that each and every item listed here has a use. For example: I'll bet you didn't know that the very first thing you should do when faced with a bloodstain is to scrape as much of it off as you can with a blunt kitchen knife; wiping usually only serves to smear the material even deeper into the fabric. Plus, you likely didn't realize that many products not exactly meant for clothes (such as 3 percent hydrogen peroxide, baby powder, and waterless mechanic's soap) can actually work wonders on some of the world's most common stains. I've compiled a handy list of the top fourteen things people always manage to stain their clothes with on page 219, so flip ahead and check them out if you're a stain-prone diva yourself. I see you there, getting grass satins on your shorts while sitting on the ground at a music festival (or dripping ketchup onto your favorite white dress while eating a hot dog in front of a bar at midnight), and I've got you covered.

THE NUCLEAR STAIN-REMOVAL OPTIONS

I can't believe I'm suggesting this, but if you are feeling particularly adventurous, it's possible to purchase professional dry-cleaning fluid online. It works like absolutely nothing else to remove stains—especially greasy, oily ones from items that absolutely cannot get wet. It's an almost-last-resort option after all other stain removers have failed. (And if even dry-cleaning fluid doesn't work to remove your stain, there's one more last-ditch option to solve a stubborn stain problem at the very end of this chapter.) I use professional dry-cleaning fluid at work only when an actor has stained clothes beyond help and all hope is truly lost.

But beware: Dry-cleaning fluid is crazy toxic—and it can be too easy to have it go wrong, fast. If you choose to take the plunge, only use it in a well-ventilated area, preferably outdoors. Always wear gloves, don't get any on your skin, and avoid breathing the fumes directly. (I wear a paper painter's face mask or a respirator when I use it.)

Now that I've sufficiently scared you, I'll tell you how to use it. Place a wad of paper towels or an absorbent cloth under your stained garment and apply the dry-cleaning fluid directly to the stain in miniscule amounts with a glass eyedropper. Do not allow any plastic objects to come into contact with the fluid—it can eat through plastic with alarming ease. Blot excess fluid firmly and carefully with another wad of paper towels until the stain disappears.

Once the stain is completely gone, toss your soiled paper towels in an outdoor trash can and blot the area with a slightly damp cloth. Finally, dry your garment completely with a hair dryer on low heat to prevent leaving a "ring" where the fluid was. Thoroughly rinse your gloves, work area, eyedropper, and any other tools immediately after you've used them.

Never attempt to treat suede, leather, or fur on your own at home— even some professional dry cleaners won't tackle these items! I use dry-cleaning fluid for stain removal only—never, ever in an attempt to perform at-home dry-cleaning. And don't put anything you've treated with dry-cleaning fluid in the dryer—it is incredibly flammable. If you want the bang of dry-cleaning fluid without all the risk, the stain-removal systems that come with at-home dry-cleaning kits actually perform pretty well with far less toxicity.

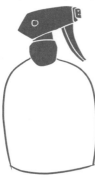
If water, soap, store-bought remedies, all my secret fixes, and even dry-cleaning fluid have failed (or you've accidentally heat-dried a terrible, impenetrable stain), you still have one last-ditch option to attempt its removal. It's a total last resort, but treating set-in stains with a dry solvent like mineral spirits (a common paint thinner, available at your local hardware store) sometimes works. (You can also use

a little WD-40, which contains a small amount of mineral spirits but is far less toxic than the real thing.) But if something catches on fire, don't say I didn't warn you: mineral spirits are highly flammable and should only be used in a well-ventilated area while wearing gloves and a mask or respirator.

Using the edge of a clean cloth that has been soaked in mineral spirits, apply the fluid directly to the stain sparingly until the stain starts to lighten. Once the stain is almost completely gone, rinse with a bit of rubbing alcohol to finish breaking down the stain and then launder your item promptly. Do not use mineral spirits or WD40 on any delicate fabric such as rayon, acetate, or 100 percent polyester— it will cause these fabrics to melt and sizzle right before your eyes, like a child's science experiment gone horribly wrong. Denim, linen, and fabrics that contain at least 50 percent cotton fare best with this method. There is always a slight chance that treating a stain with solvents will result in a small "ring" where the stain was. This is most likely due to the migration of the dye in the fabric when you dissolved your stain, and it's never going to go away. So there is obviously a fair amount of risk involved in attempting this stain solution—that's why it's the true, final, nuclear option, only to be attempted when all else has failed. It should be reserved solely for items that are otherwise destined for the trash.

WHEN ALL ELSE FAILS, JUST DYE IT!

If even using mineral spirits doesn't work to remove your stain, you might want to consider overdyeing the garment another color (one that's darker than the stain). I use regular old Rit Dye in my home washer, taking care to clean my machine thoroughly afterward. If you have a new-fangled, high-efficiency front-loading washer, you might be less than pleased with the outcome—less water means a smaller dye bath. If you find the results aren't so stellar, just ditch the washer altogether and dye your garments in a bucket with some hot water from the kettle.

Dyeing clothes doesn't always work out, but I've had a decent amount of happy accidents that resulted in something I thought was dead getting a new lease on life after having a relaxing soak in a dye bath. However, I've also had my share of dyeing disasters that ended with the item hitting the dustbin—but that's where a terribly stained garment was most likely headed anyway, so you've really got nothing to lose! Dyeing works best on 100 percent cotton, linen, silk, and synthetics like rayon and nylon. (Polyester is a synthetic fabric as well but won't take regular Rit Dye no matter what you do. I know this because my attempt to dye a polyester garment is how I ended up with a dress bubbling away on my stove way back when I met the first director to ever give me a costume design job!) Always use the hottest water you can, and never dump the dye directly onto your clothing. Whether you are using liquid or powder dye, allow it to dissolve in water completely before adding your garments to the mix—otherwise, the dye is likely to spot and leave a speckled pattern on your clothes.

Adding a tablespoon of laundry soap and a cup of salt to the dye bath after your garments have been soaking for about five minutes will help to lock in a more intense color. And a cup of white vinegar (which you now have handy in your stain kit, right?) also helps to amp up the color when dyeing silk or nylon fabrics. Treat your dyed pieces as hand-washables—just like we talked about earlier in this chapter. See how this is all coming together? Slowly but surely, I'm turning you into someone who cares about taking good care of your clothes. I'll bet you don't even recognize yourself.

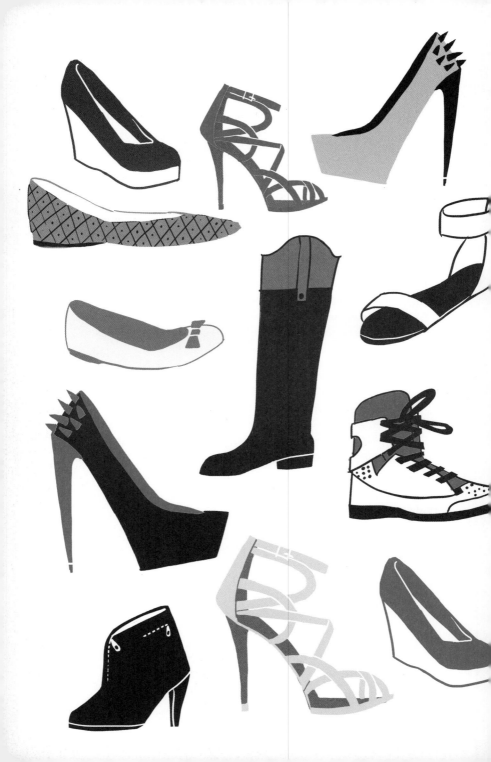

CHAPTER 11

SHOE CARE
for all your footwear

Let's pause for a moment so I can make a confession: I don't take very good care of my actors' shoes. I kind of don't have to! They only wear them for short periods of time and almost always on a nice, temperature-controlled soundstage. There's someone standing by with their slippers between takes, and if they have to walk very far, someone just takes them in a golf cart. As a result, I do almost zero work to maintain their footwear. The only time I actually bother to clean actors' shoes is if they've just been involved in an on-camera food fight, something that happens a little too often when you are the costume designer on a kid's show. (If you're considering going to school for a degree in costume design, keep the image of me scrubbing cake and spaghetti out of shoes in the on-stage toilets fresh in your mind as you study.)

My personal shoes, however, are a different story. I exclusively wear boots to work, and they are usually of the several-hundred-dollar variety. So I make it a point to take excellent care of them—because a well-made pair of leather shoes or boots can fend off an attack of mold, being caught in a sudden downpour, or having stinky, sweaty feet shoved into them constantly and keep on truckin' for years to come. You just need to give them a little TLC every now and then! Your best bet is obviously to prevent problems before they start, so here are the preventative shoe-care tips I use in my own closet, plus some advice as to what you can do to salvage your footwear if a shoe tragedy has already struck (in addition to a few tricks to make a painful pair just a little more tolerable). And PS: Almost all the advice here easily can be adapted to care for your leather and suede handbags, too!

HELP YOUR SHOES KEEP THEIR SHAPE

The best thing you can do for your favorite shoes is to always use a shoe tree when you aren't actively wearing them. What sounds like a crazy luxury meant only for rich bankers is actually a smart invest-ment; shoes that maintain their shape live longer, happier lives. Daily shoe-tree use prevents the leather from curling and cracking, as the shoe's shape is maintained by the tension of the tree. (It also helps lessen creasing across the toe.) There are endless styles of shoe trees available, including ones meant for heels, boots, and lace-ups, in addition to inflatable versions perfect for traveling. I am partial to the classic cedar shoe tree; a well-made set can last a lifetime with periodic sanding to reactivate the cedar. I've got a few that actually belonged to my grandfather! While it may seem that shoe trees should be reserved for use in only your most expensive footwear, even cheaper, lesser-quality shoes can benefit from using them. Trees keep your shoe's toe box and heel structures from falling and being crushed, causing them to look better when they are on your foot and waltzing down the street.

Still not convinced? Consider this: During a normal day, your feet produce a disgusting one-quarter cup of moisture, also known as foot sweat. A cedar shoe tree acts as a natural deodorant—and helps to draw that moisture out of your shoes and prevent the leather from wrinkling and cracking as a result of being rode hard and put away wet. (You can also just use some tightly packed newspaper to dry out a pair of sweaty shoes in a pinch.)

SPRING FOR PROTECTIVE RUBBER SOLES— AND REPLACE YOUR HEEL CAPS OFTEN

If your shoes have leather soles, your very first order of business (even before wearing them out to dinner) should be to take them to a shoe repair shop and ask to have ultra-thin rubber soles put on. (Some shops call it dance rubber.) When done right, this protective covering is invisible from the side, provides extra traction when you are walking, and extends the life of your shoes almost indefinitely. Not sure if your shoes have leather soles? If you paid more than $200 for them, chances are they have leather soles. The paradox here is that the more expensive the shoe, the more fragile the sole. A well-crafted leather sole is a sign of a quality shoe—but it can also lead to the shoe's early demise if it's not properly protected. A good rubber-sole application should run you about $25 a pair—and after you do it once, you'll retroactively mourn all the beautiful shoes you had that wore out early because you didn't care enough to do this for them.

Another thing to pay careful attention to is your heels. If you've ever been walking in a pair of stilettos and noticed they were making a metallic clicking sound when your heel struck the ground, it was most likely because you wore the original heel cap down to the bare metal spike inside. Once that spike is exposed, you are grinding it down with every step you take. The only permanent solution is having your heel tips replaced by a cobbler, but you can temporarily keep them going for a few more wears with some store-bought adhesive heel caps. Whatever you do, do not keep walking once metal is exposed! By doing so, you are causing serious damage to the heel itself—and increasing your chances of slipping and falling on polished floors.

REMOVE SALT AND SLUSH RESIDUE IMMEDIATELY

Any time your shoes are exposed to salt and slush, permanent damage is occurring with every step. Salt is enemy number one of leather: It starts corroding your shoes the minute it makes contact. Get into the habit of wiping any accumulated salt residue from your shoes as soon as possible with a slightly damp rag moistened with a mixture of plain white vinegar and warm water. At the very least, make it a point to use a dry cloth to wipe your shoes down after walking in inclement weather. I carry a clean cloth diaper in my bag when I wear my good boots anywhere it snows. I sometimes get funny looks from security guards, but it's well worth it—because this one simple act can save your footwear from certain element-inflicted demise.

AVOID HEAT AND OTHER DRYING CONDITIONS

Never dry your leather shoes anywhere near a heater or using a hair dryer. Excessive heat causes leather to dry out, crack, and become brittle. Your best bet is to allow your shoes to air-dry with newspaper stuffed into the toes. You can speed the process up a little by using a fan—or investing in an electric shoe dryer like we use on set. (You'd barf out of your eyes if you saw how sopping wet and sweaty an actor's shoes can get after a single day of filming.) An electric shoe dryer is a miracle gadget—it can take a pair of shoes from sopping wet to bone dry overnight. They cost anywhere from $30 to $100, and if you live anywhere that sees lots of rain or snow, it's a smart investment.

ROTATE YOUR FOOTWEAR

Just like you, your shoes need a day off now and then. Giving them a break after wearing them for two consecutive days allows them to fully dry out—and dry shoes obviously aren't able to retain moisture and odors. Letting your shoes rest in between wearings also helps them keep their shape and not get hopelessly stretched out.

DON'T FORGET TO WATERPROOF

Leather shoes plus bad weather is a deadly combination, so before you wear them out in the slush or rain, make sure you waterproof them. But the term "waterproofing" is a bit of a misnomer, as all you are really doing is improving their ability to withstand water. No spray can really make a leather shoe completely impervious to rain and water. I prefer new-fangled, silicone-based waterproofing sprays instead of the old classic mink oil because oil-based waterproofers can darken leather.

Whatever waterproofing product you decide to use, take the time to test an inconspicuous corner of your shoes for any possible color change. If the shoes are made of suede, be sure to choose a waterproofing product specifically meant for use on suede. The nap (or raised surface) of suede shoes is easily disturbed and ruined, so a product that works on smooth leather is unsuitable.

Waterproofing your leather shoes or boots is only half the battle. Allowing all-leather shoes to air-dry properly after use in a damp environment is of the utmost importance. Just be careful how you dry them—and remember to never, ever use heat. If you are putting your leather shoes away for the season, go the extra mile and pack them with a moisture-absorbing desiccant sachet—which is what comes in those mini-packets that new shoes and handbags are packaged with that you aren't supposed to eat!

Larger, premade desiccant sachets do exist, but you can also just make your own for cheap by using an old sock and a box of "crystal" cat litter. (Crystal cat litter is made of pure silica gel crystals, the exact same ingredient found in ready-made desiccant sachets.) Simply fill the sock toe with cat litter and secure the end by tying it in a knot or wrapping it with a rubber band, leaving enough space to allow the sachet to mold itself to the shape of your shoes. For about $8, you can make forty or more sachets—and share them with friends! Now, aren't you glad you bought a book written by a girl who likes to look good on the cheap?

MAINTAIN, MAINTAIN, MAINTAIN

To keep your smooth leather boots clean, shiny, and scuff-free, it's a good idea to treat yourself to a shoeshine every now and then. The old-fashioned shoeshine booth does still exist—you can usually find one located anywhere businessmen tend to congregate, like airports. So hop on up in the chair with a newspaper and chill out like a character in an old-timey movie. You can obviously shine your shoes yourself, but after watching my dad spit shine his shoes Army-style for years, I can assure you that it's a hell of a lot of hard work. If you are so inclined, here are his basic steps: clean, condition, and polish.

CLEAN

Yes, you should be cleaning your shoes on a regular basis—but the cleaning method is dependent on the shoe's material. In most cases, a simple wipe with a clean rag or a brisk brushing with a soft shoe brush will suffice. For smooth leather shoes, you can use a store-bought leather cleaner or just a clean rag dampened with a little white vinegar and warm water. If your shoes are *really* dirty, use saddle soap and water for deeper, more thorough cleaning. Saddle soap is available at most auto-supply stores, and the best application method is to use a clean, damp cloth or a soft bristled brush (like horsehair), working some of the soap onto the cloth until you create a nice lather. Then apply the lather to the shoes while rubbing gently. Be sure to wipe down leather items cleaned with saddle soap thoroughly with a slightly damp rag; the residue can damage leather—just like dried soap left on your skin will. And never, ever use any cleaner containing detergent, which can easily destroy leather's natural oils.

Patent leather shoes have been treated with a lacquer to give them that high-gloss shine—and it also makes them relatively easy to care for. A brisk swish with a lint-free cloth is all most patent shoes will ever need, and minor scuffs can be removed easily with a cotton swab dipped in rubbing alcohol or mineral oil. For more stubborn marks, you can use a pencil eraser (a gum eraser is best) to gently "erase" the scuffs through friction. An actor I once worked with on a military drama swore by the power of a slice of white bread to remove scuffs from patent leather. I guess it's meant to act as a sponge? Since he wore shiny patent dress shoes as part of his costume every day, I decided to try it—and I'm sad to report that it actually does not work at all. Also, heat can cause patent leather shoes to stick to each other, so wrap them in an old towel or T-shirt before storing for an extended period of time.

For suede shoes, steam from a fabric iron or your trusty hand steamer held about ten inches away from the shoe and a good brushing with a stiff-bristle brush (like a clean toothbrush) or a suede bar is an excellent way to remove stains and dirt. Always brush in the direction of the fibers, unless you have caked in dirt or mud. If scuff marks remain after brushing, you can attempt their removal with a suede eraser (sold at most drugstores) or even an emery board. Never brush suede shoes when wet—it only succeeds in spreading the dirt further into the shoe's surface. Some shoe care experts swear by a wire-bristled brush to restore the nap to suede shoes, but I think it's far too easy to rip and shred your shoes with one.

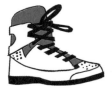 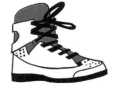

Fabric shoes are a little more difficult to clean and should be sprayed with a good stain guard (such as Scotchgard, available at any store that carries shoe-care supplies) before wearing. A quick application of stain guard now will save you heartache later when someone pours a glass of red wine on your wedding shoes, and it's also brilliant at keeping your canvas sneakers looking newer longer. Just spray it on your shoes in light, even strokes in a well-ventilated area and allow them to dry thoroughly before wearing.

To remove grime or soil from fabric shoes, give them a good brushing with a soft-bristle brush lightly coated with baking soda, then hand wash inside a tied-up pillowcase in a sink full of cool water and a bit of color-safe detergent. Rinse thoroughly and allow to fully air-dry before wearing. You can also give them a spin in the washer (again, inside a pillowcase) with your machine set to gentle—just toss a few towels in to protect your shoes from getting banged around. Never put fabric shoes in the dryer, and always allow them to air-dry fully before wearing, because the fibers will stretch out and fray if pressure is applied when wet.

If you've got a pair of nonleather or pleather (also known as vinyl) shoes, care and cleaning is totally easy—because it's really a form of plastic! Regular wiping with a damp rag and a bit of warm soapy water will keep dirt and grime at bay, and most scuffs can easily be removed with Windex and a paper towel. For more serious scuffs, use a gum eraser in a back-and-forth motion until the scuffs are no longer visible. Never use any harsh cleaners or solvents (such as acetone) on a nonleather shoe, as it can remove or damage the protective coating. If you've got marks that just won't budge, you can give your item new life with a can of aerosol vinyl "dye" coating (available at better shoe repair shops). It will eventually begin to chip and flake, but it's a good way to get a few more wearings out of your nonleather goods.

CONDITION

After cleaning your leather shoes, it's a good idea to apply a lanolin-based conditioner such as Lexol brand leather conditioner. It will help to replace the leather's natural oils, which can get lost with daily wear. While your shoes are still slightly damp from cleaning, apply the product in a circular motion with a clean, dry cloth. Set your clean, conditioned shoes aside for a good twenty-four hours so they can dry completely. (PS: The drying process is a good time to use your shoe trees! As you already know, they help your shoes dry evenly and retain their shape.)

POLISH

Always use a paste or cream polish to shine your smooth leather shoes. Waxes, liquid polish, and "instant shine" sponges will indeed give a super-fast, high-shine finish to your shoes, but they are drying and can crack the leather over time. Cream and paste polishes help to moisturize leather while keeping it flexible. Make sure the polish you choose matches the shoes, and use one shade lighter than the leather color to cover scratches. (Oh, and psssst!

Neutral polish is your go-to for light-colored shoes.) Apply the polish with a clean, soft, slightly damp rag (like a pair of old socks), wrapping the cloth around your first two fingers and twisting the remainder of the cloth into the palm of your hand. Cover the entire shoe with a generous amount of polish, taking care to get down every seam of the shoe. (And add a little more dampness to the rag as you go if you are looking to get a true "mirror shine" for your footwear!) Allow the polish to dry for ten to fifteen minutes, then buff it off with a horsehair polishing brush, leaving only a small film on the shoes. Lastly, give your shoes a brisk buff with a soft, clean cloth to bring out their original luster.

BRING YOUR SHOES BACK FROM THE DEAD

What about when preventative maintenance has failed, and you think a pair of shoes is too far gone to save? Read on before you toss something that could actually be saved—because it's quite possible to revive almost any shoe, no matter what terrible tragedy has befallen it.

RAIN-DAMAGED, MOLDY, OR WET SHOES

Sometimes, despite your best efforts to keep your leather shoes warm and dry, the unthinkable can still happen: mold. If you notice a powdery white substance taking up residence on your shoes, chances are it's a little bit of dastardly mold. A good firm brushing with a stiff nylon brush (you can use a kitchen or nail brush if you like) will usually remove most—if not all—of the mold immediately.

But if some still remains, your next step is to carefully wipe the affected areas with a well-wrung rag dampened with a mixture of equal parts white vinegar and water—vinegar is a natural fungicide. Just make sure you don't allow the leather surface to become completely soaking wet—a slightly damp application is all you are aiming for. You can also use the same damp rag method with a water-diluted mixture of rubbing alcohol or tea tree oil to kill and remove stubborn mold.

(The ratio should be one-half cup of water to five or six drops of full-strength tea tree oil or one-half cup of water to one-quarter cup rubbing alcohol.)

Make sure to allow the shoes you've treated to dry thoroughly afterward. A caveat: If you have a mold problem on suede, I wouldn't recommend using vinegar or any other wet fluid on them. Your best bet is to invest in a good suede brush, give 'em a brisk brushing, and then leave them outside in full sun. (Sunshine is a natural mold killer.) If you've got a really tough mold situation, a spot cleaning with a brass-bristled suede brush can help remove it, but be as gentle as possible—and never use a brass brush on light-colored suede or nubuck.

After removing the mold, you may want to give your smooth leather shoes or boots a good washing with some mild saddle soap (as discussed on page 173) if they appear dirty or grimy. I find saddle soap especially useful to remove salt stains from leather. But proceed with great care—an improper washing with saddle soap can do more harm than good. If your boots aren't dirty or stained, skip this step completely. Again, take care to never allow the leather to become soaking wet— just work the saddle soap into a lather using a clean, damp cloth or a soft-bristled shoe brush (like a horsehair one), buffing in a circular motion to work out the stains. Then wipe the soap off with a soft, damp cloth, repeating as necessary to remove all sticky residue.

Anytime you apply liquid to a leather hide, a proper conditioning treatment is a must. Just like your skin, leather gets dried out after any contact with water—rain included. You can combat this problem by regularly using a high-quality leather conditioner to renew your leather's natural oils. Luckily, leather conditioners come in a handy-wipe version, which is a super-easy delivery system, but if you choose to go the liquid route, rub it in carefully with a clean, soft, dry cloth. (And in case you missed it before: Cotton cloth diapers are the gold standard for shoe care.)

You may find that even after all this effort, you're left with a pair of leather shoes that looks less than stellar. But that's the beauty of buying quality leather goods—they really do have nine lives. To bring well-worn or permanently stained leather shoes back to life, send them to your favorite shoe repair spot for a professional dye job—a bottle of dye hides a multitude of sins. This is also a great tip if you have boots or shoes in a color you detest. My favorite shoe dude successfully dyed a pair of boots that were once a boring light gray to a blazing hot pink color, much to the delight of my pal who was about to put them in a donation bin. Dyeing leather shoes on your own is, in my opinion, a fool's errand. I've absolutely never had it turn out right, so it's well worth the money to have a professional do it for you.

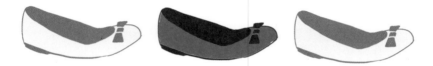

SWEATY, SMELLY, STINKY SHOES

Here's the best reader question I think I've ever received: "Hey Alison, any idea of what you can do about a really stinky, swampy, smelly shoe?" After I stopped laughing, I realized that I've actually been a victim of this dreadful foot stank myself—and I think I know why. I wear a lot of tights with sneakers or boots as part of my everyday work look, and most tights don't have any cotton content—at least not enough to absorb sweat and odor. So all that foot sweat is going straight into the insole of my shoes—and it can smell really bad. As it turns out, the simple act of switching your socks is likely the answer to your foot stink problems. All cotton socks are good—but those fancy microfiber socks that wick moisture away from your feet are even better, because any sock that traps sweat (like an all-nylon one) can easily lead to rampant shoe stink. I've started wearing socks either under or over my tights, both to absorb sweat and to make them less prone to running and tearing in the toe and foot.

A smelly shoe problem is made even worse when you truly love a pair of shoes and wear them multiple days in a row—because they don't get a chance to dry out and de-stink themselves, so your foot funk has an opportunity to build up and become terrible. Shoes that are made from pleather or rubber can also be the culprit—they don't allow the foot to breathe, thereby trapping sweaty stink inside with no place to go. And you might be surprised that simply not allowing your feet to dry completely after showering and before putting on your shoes can result in some seriously rank foot odor. That little bit of water left trapped between your toes can be slow to dry and quick to funkify.

To combat the shoe stink even more, make sure to allow your shoes to dry out completely between wearings. This can be helped along by stuffing newspaper inside each shoe to absorb the excess moisture that's left behind. You can also make your own moisture absorbing inserts by filling a pair of old socks with either activated charcoal (like they use in home aquariums, available at most pet stores) or plain old baking soda. (Both can be messy to work with, so don't just rip the package open and start pouring it into your spare socks all willy-nilly!) While silica crystal sachets (like the homemade cat litter versions we talked about making back on page 172) are a good choice for combating moisture when putting your shoes away for the season, baking soda or charcoal versions are what you need if you're fighting foot stink. Stuff your homemade absorbent sachets in each shoe after every single wearing. If you do it religiously, it will keep the stink far, far away.

Tapping a little baby or foot powder in your shoes before each wearing also makes a huge difference in soaking up odor. But once a stank-foot smell has taken up seemingly permanent residence, what can you do to get rid of it? The solution lies in a pretty simple concept—killing the bacteria that causes the stink. If it's a pair of washable sneakers, a spin through the washer in hot water with a tiny capful of well-diluted bleach usually does the trick. But a pair of leather shoes is a different story. To de-funk a nonwashable shoe fast, try running a cotton ball soaked with either rubbing alcohol or Pine Sol all over the inside of the shoe and insole, allowing it to dry completely before wearing. You may need to do this twice, but it really is great at neutralizing stink on the double. Leaving the offending shoes outside in bright sunlight will also work to kill the odor—as sunshine is an all-natural, surprisingly effective disinfectant. (You'll be shocked at just how well sunshine really works, I promise—so be sure to try it.) If you want to de-funk your footwear like rock stars do, crib this trick I learned while on the road with a band, where I was tasked with keeping their all-leather stage wear free from the stink of thousands of adoring fans: Get yourself some vodka, the cheapest kind you can, and pour it undiluted into a spray bottle. Spritz freely and wipe down any surface with it that smells bad—the ethanol in the booze "naturally" disinfects and deodorizes leather clothing and shoes like nothing else. (And if you need to make sure the nozzle on your spray bottle is working properly, you can just give your mouth a few squirts as a little "test.") Vodka dries almost instantly and doesn't leave your leather items soaking wet. If you suspect your smelly socks are what's causing your shoe stink, vodka is the cure for them, too. Give them a relaxing soak in a 50 percent vodka/50 percent water solution for about an hour and then launder as usual.

A spritz of classic Lysol spray also never fails to eradicate shoe stench—but if you want to de-stink your shoes like wardrobe girls do, grab a can of what bowling alleys have used for ages to kill the funk of a thousand feet: End Bac II disinfectant spray, available online at Manhattan Wardrobe Supply and at most office supply stores. It's a germicide spray that kills fungus, mold, mildew, and even the bacteria that causes tuberculosis. One spritz ends foot funk forever. (Just be sure to use it in a well-ventilated area; it has a rather strong chemical odor.)

FLAPPING SHOE SOLES

If the soles of your shoes have come undone, don't waste your time and money going to a proper shoe repair spot—instead, spend $7 on a tube of Shoe Goo, the liquid "rubber in a tube." It's available at most hardware stores, and I've used it for many questionable repairs to some rather expensive shoes that have lasted for years. Just be sure to use it in a well-ventilated area; apply it in a thin, even layer using a popsicle stick; and allow it to cure for a full twenty-four hours before wearing your shoes.

KEEP YOUR SHOES FROM KILLING YOUR FEET

But what about the "ouch" factor? It doesn't matter how much money you pay for a pair of shoes, they will likely wind up hurting your feet in some terrible way. I have outrageously expensive shoes that chafe, rub, and destroy my tootsies. I also have cheap shoes that fit like a dream! There just isn't a way to definitively tell if a shoe is going to be good to you until you are suddenly very far from home, hobbling along the streets as your feet are being cut to ribbons. But whatever your foot drama, chances are I've got a solution to your problem right here.

IF YOUR SHOES ARE TOO TIGHT

If your leather shoes are just a hair too tight, you can sometimes stretch them at home using plain old rubbing alcohol (also known as isopropyl alcohol). Wear a pair of rubber gloves for protection and dip your fingers into the alcohol, massaging and kneading the part of the shoe that needs to be stretched for a few minutes. You want it saturated—not soaked.

After working the area you want stretched, put the shoes on with the thickest pair of socks you can find and wear them around the house for a few hours. I usually try this at-home method first, before springing for professional shoe stretching. If your too-small shoes are made of fabric, I've got bad news—stretching them almost never works. It puts too much pressure on the fibers, causing them to snap and break.

IF YOUR SHOES ARE CHAFING, RUBBING, OR CAUSING BLISTERS

The foolproof solution for shoes that dig, rub, cut, blister, and chafe your feet is self-adhesive moleskin, which is readily available in the foot care aisle of every drugstore. (See pages 80–82 for more on the wonders of this miracle product.) The common misconception is that moleskin is meant to be applied to your skin—but really, sticking it directly to the shoe itself is the answer to almost all foot pain. Just cut it to the desired shape and line anywhere inside the shoe that is rubbing your foot raw.

If you are prone to getting blisters, the likely culprit is friction. Cut the friction, and you'll cut the blisters. For my fancy actors, I often buy a friction block stick from the drugstore foot-care aisle to form an invisible barrier on their feet that reduces rubbing—ergo, reducing blisters. But for myself at home, I sometimes just use the tiniest bit of Crisco vegetable shortening or nonstick cooking spray to achieve the same lubricating effect (see page 85). (Good ol' Vaseline works pretty well, too!)

IF YOUR TOES ARE CRUSHED, YOU MIGHT BE GETTING BUNIONS

Right now, as you read this, if you happen to be wearing shoes, you're probably ruining your feet. And it's because almost every shoe on the market, flat or heeled, has a toe box design that is too small and tapered to allow your toes to be properly aligned. The result? Foot deformity—and painful bunions. If a bump is starting to appear on the outside of your big toe, and you see that toe is beginning to point toward your second toe, it's quite likely that you're on the road to bunions—and it's not a fun journey. How do I know? I'm walking that road myself.

Bunions occur when the taper of a shoe's toe box begins right where your foot is actually at it's widest. The pressure forces your toe joints to drift inward, causing a bony lump to form on the outside of your big toe—and sometimes even on your little toe. (The little toe bunion is commonly called a bunionette, which sounds totally adorable until you realize how painful one is.) Some bunions are totally hereditary—and no type of shoe can save those peeps from getting them. Growing up without shoes is the best way to avoid getting bunions, but other than that, you can keep them at bay by always making sure you can wiggle and separate your toes inside your shoes freely—because if you can't, chances are those shoes are totally ruining your feet. Using the wiggle-room rule, most of my favorite shoes are out. Even some of my sneakers don't pass this test! It's a sad truth, but most shoes available for purchase these days are too narrow—and cram your toes together unnaturally, causing them to overlap, allowing painful bunions to start forming. The only way to attempt to "cure" bunions is surgery, which doesn't always work—and many times, the bunions return. So I got rid of a shocking dollar amount of fancy shoes and never looked back. As a result, my bunions haven't gotten any worse. In addition to only buying shoes with enough wiggle room, I've also had some luck using toe spacers to gently realign my toes after the times I break down and wear a pair of shoes that I really shouldn't be wearing—because I'm not yet at the point where I can bring myself to wear Birkenstocks to a wedding.

IF YOUR SHOES ARE TOO BIG OR THE BALLS OF YOUR FEET ARE ALWAYS BURNING

I keep a variety of implements in my costuming kit to make actors' shoes fit better, but I use only two of them over and over: heel grips and ball-of-foot pads. A silicone or suede self-adhesive heel grip is a game-changer if you've endured a lifetime of heel slippage in shoes. And that burning sensation under the ball of your foot? Banish it forever with a puffy, stick-in pad meant to provide extra cushioning while you walk. Some better shoe stores stock and will provide them free with purchase—you just have to ask.

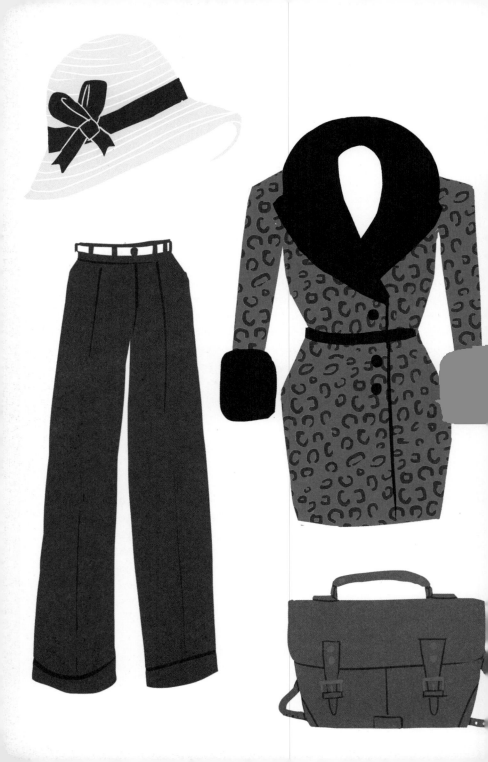

CHAPTER 12

OLD STUFF:
a guide to shopping vintage and thrift

Have you ever complimented a pal on something they're wearing, only to have them say, "Thanks! It's vintage!" (and/or from the thrift store) and wondered, "How come I can never find anything like that when I look?" Shopping vintage is paradoxically both harder and easier than it seems. I actually do a fair amount of thrift and vintage shopping on small, low, or no-budget productions, but I also hit up my local secondhand spot even when I have a generous amount of money to work with on a show. Sometimes it's because a particular character's look demands it—but more often than not, I go simply because the variety is endless. Instead of the sea of sameness at the local mall, there is excitement in never quite knowing what you're going to find. I happen to love a good scavenger hunt—but even if you don't, thrift and vintage shopping is an excellent way to stretch your clothing budget. You just have to know how to do it right! I've got some tips on how to do it like a pro, but first, let's discuss the differences between the various types of establishments that sell secondhand fashion.

THRIFT STORES AND CHARITY SHOPS

A true thrift store is a place where almost no clothing or accessory item is over $20. They tend to be rather disorganized, and it takes a lot of digging to find the one single, stellar piece in a football fields' worth of lesser garments. You might think that all thrift stores are created equal as they run on donations, but this isn't always true. Many big-name thrift stores are actually for-profit enterprises. I always go out of my way to frequent "charity" shops run by churches, schools, and women's organizations instead. They usually have a "boutique" feel—which is a direct result of being run by dedicated volunteers who get their donations from affluent communities, resulting in better-quality items for sale than at your average thrift store (but for very close to the same prices). Entire estates sometimes get donated to charity shops, resulting in some stellar finds.

VINTAGE STORES

A true vintage store is not a cheap affair. They are usually run by collectors with heaps of knowledge about vintage fashion, and you're not likely to find anything for sale in one for less than about $50—and prices can spike upward of $1,000. These stores always carry at least a handful of "collectible" and "designer" pieces from various eras—with the prices to match. There are plenty of spots out there looking to cash in on the vintage craze, attempting to sell you items of dubious quality just because they happen to be old. Not all old things are necessarily good things, so never was the phrase "buyer beware" more apropos than when shopping for high-end vintage.

CONSIGNMENT OR RESALE SHOPS

Consignment shops differ from thrift, charity, and vintage stores because they function as a reselling agent for a seller who wishes to unload clothes, shoes, or accessories. In the consignment scenario, an individual seller brings goods to the store and agrees to leave them there until they are sold or the contract between the store and seller is up. The store typically keeps anywhere from 40 to 50 percent of the sale as a commission. Consignment is usually reserved for higher-end fashions and is an excellent purchasing resource if you are a fan of ultrafancy designer brands and styles. Expect to pay about half to a quarter of the original retail price for name-brand goods in a consignment store.

USED CLOTHING STORES

In recent years, outlets dedicated to the buying and selling of used, trendy clothing have sprung up far and wide. If you are doing a closet cleanout and have stylish, good-condition garments to unload, consider making back a bit of their purchase price by selling them to a used clothing store. You'll walk away with about 20 percent of each item's selling price in cash, but items can have absolutely no stains, holes, rips, or tears to be accepted. Prices in a used clothing store are, on average, higher than a thrift store or charity shop—but still far less than the original retail cost. Better used clothing stores will post buying hours prominently, along with the styles they are currently buying. It's a great way to recycle your clothes, make a little money, and pick up some "new-to-you" pieces all in one fell swoop.

TO START THE HUNT, PREPARE AND PLAN

Part of the reason people don't have success shopping in vintage or thrift stores is because they just pop into any old random spot the very first time and quickly scan the racks, deem it all gross, and move on. (This was totally me the first time I tried!) But proper preparation is essential to a successful hunt. I like to start by giving my closet a once-over to see what I'm lacking and what I already have too many of—because if I already have fifty-seven floral dresses that I wear and love, number fifty-eight isn't going to get a lot of play in the rotation, so I probably shouldn't bring it home. I also do a quick browse of the top mainstream fast-fashion chains to see what looks they are currently pushing—it puts fresh ideas in my mind and those items then instantly pop into my line of vision when I'm out searching.

To ensure a successful shopping trip, it helps to wear something smart. Flat shoes are a must, as there is lots of walking involved in an after-noon of hitting vintage and thrift stores. Wear shoes that are simple to slip on and off, and pack a pair of thin socks in your bag even if you don't usually wear them. You'll thank me later when you're not stand-ing barefoot on a dirty floor. Also, make sure to dress in something that allows you to try things on over your clothes, like a tank top and leggings, in case a dressing room isn't available.

Carry a purse that allows you to work hands free. (I swear by a small cross-body style.) Then, pack it with a handful of secondhand shopping essentials: hand wipes for banishing after-shopping grossness, tissues in case of dust allergies, a small stain remover pen to check if a spot has any hope of coming out, and a fabric tape measure. (That tape measure will become your new best friend once I teach you how to take your basic measurements toward the end of this chapter, because when you know your measurements, you'll never have to actually try on clothes again if you don't want to!) I also like to bring a reusable grocery sack to stuff all my items in while I shop—as a cart or basket left unattended at the end of an aisle is ripe for nosey hands to dig into.

THEN, KNOW WHAT TO LOOK FOR

To be a great shopper, you need to become a label whore! Educating yourself about well-known and little-known fashion designers alike is one of the best ways to become a better vintage and thrift shopper. The Vintage Fashion Guild's comprehensive "Label Resource" (vintagefashionguild.com) is an excellent way to learn more about designers and their labels so you can start to spot them in the store. While there are too many vintage designers for the average shopper to ever remember, a good rule of thumb is the more intricate the label, the higher the likelihood that it's an actual vintage piece. Another reliable way to spot classic vintage pieces is to look for the "Union Made" label—specifically that of the International Ladies' Garment Workers' Union, or ILGWU. (It may also say "AFL-CIO" on it, which is the mark of the American Federation of Labor and Congress of Industrial Organizations.) If a garment has the "Union Made" tag sewn inside, you are almost guaranteed that it's at least twenty years old—because beginning in the 1980s, overseas manufacturing began chipping away at the ILGWU. By 1995, the union was completely dissolved.

It also helps to know your eras. Modern designers reference styles from years gone by all the time—and being able to quickly identify these vintage-inspired shapes is a great way to determine if a piece is worth picking up or not. People go to school for years to learn about every decade's fashion touchstones, but you can become a back-pocket expert just by referring to the handy cheat sheet below while shopping. (Oh—and for the record, vintage is usually classified as being at least twenty-five years old—anything pre-1920 is classified as an antique.) Keep in mind that the earlier the decade, the harder it is to find an actual, authentic vintage piece for sale at any price—time is not always kind to fabric, and many pieces available from high-end vintage sellers aren't meant to be worn as they are far too fragile. But knowing how to spot a good reproduction or "vintage-inspired" piece when they happen to pop up is invaluable. (Otherwise, you'll never know what you're missing out on!)

THE 1920S

This marked the true beginning of modern female style. Women in the United States were granted the right to vote, entered the workforce in droves, raised their hemlines, and started to assert their independence everywhere. If you currently enjoy drinking an after-work cocktail in public while wearing a short skirt, you have a flapper to thank for that! Fashions of the 1920s were a sharp contrast to the stuffy, rigid styles of the Victorian era, and jubilant embellishment was a key trend. Beaded Art Deco, Art Nouveau, and geometric designs were everywhere— along with a proliferation of decorative fringe, pleats, and slits. Loose, boyish, sporty frocks, along with drop-waist dresses, squared neck-lines, long strands of pearls, T-strap heels, and sharp Peter Pan collars are all hallmarks of Roaring Twenties style that still hold up today.

THE 1930S

Hollywood stars of the decade (and the costume designers who dressed them!) played a huge part in helping fashion veer toward ultrafeminine shapes with nipped in, defined waists and fluttery but-terfly sleeves. What was worn on the screen became the style on the streets. In 1936, legendary costume designer Edith Head put Dorothy Lamour in a tropical patterned sarong for the film *Jungle Princess*—and a year later, the sarong-style was one of the most popular looks on the beach. Slinky satin dresses were cut on the bias (meaning the fabric is cut in a diagonal direction in order to utilize it's stretch) to better accentuate the body's natural curves. Skirts grazed the anklebone, and peep-toed slingback shoes were all the rage. The 1930s was the ultimate era of old-school Hollywood glam, a look that doesn't seem out of place eighty-some-odd years later.

THE 1940S

This decade saw the meteoric rise of the practical, yet elegant shirt-dress. Usually made from printed cotton, this classic style got its name from the clever marriage of a button-front blouse to a full-skirted bottom, resulting in one totally handy garment. The shirtdress of the 1940s commonly came with a self-fabric belt or sash and was just as appropriate for doing housework as it was for running errands around town. Another totally 1940s look is the fitted, embellished knit sweater. These were often decorated with seaming, sequins, or glass beads as all spare metal was being used in the war effort. Jaunty nautical looks were another big trend toward the end of the 1940s in America as feverish patriotism swept the nation after the end of World War II. In early 1947, Christian Dior's "New Look" also helped to sweep in an era of extravagance, as the average wartime dress used just three yards of fabric—and Dior's called for no less than twenty-five. After years of doing without, women were ready for the full-skirted, full-crinoline looks that would dominate the coming decade.

THE 1950S

These years produced a veritable explosion in the styles and types of clothing available to the modern woman. While crinolines and corsets that enhanced the classic womanly shape were de rigueur, sheath dresses, pedal pushers, pencil skirts, and halter sundresses also took the decade by storm and ushered in a more modern mode of dress. The monochromatic "Beat Generation" look allowed teens to develop their own style for the first time—and saw them dressing far more casually than their parents, which served to set them apart from mainstream culture. The 1950s were also responsible for the introduction of the stiletto heel, courtesy of French shoe designer Roger Vivier.

THE 1960S

This was the "Youthquake" era, as coined by legendary *Vogue* magazine editor Diana Vreeland. For the first time in history, teens were dictating style and driving fashion design forward. Their influence on designers was unmistakable, and designers struggled to keep up with the changing tastes of this newly empowered generation. The miniskirt made its first appearance—along with the pillbox hat and that perennial classic, the Lily Pulitzer shift dress. Pop art ushered in an avalanche of wild geometric patterns (like those from Italian designer Pucci), and young women began snapping up separates to mix and match rather than wearing head-to-toe looks. Patent leather and vinyl materials reflected the dawn of the Space Age, and the race to the moon culminated in André Courrèges' 1964 "Moon Girl" collection.

THE 1970S

Hippie style began creeping onto the scene in the late 1960s but was everywhere by the early 1970s. Bell-bottom jeans, platform shoes, and romantic, peasant-style blouses are lynchpin looks of the 1970s that feel right at home even today. Tight, synthetic knit sweaters are a key 1970s style, as well as velvet tuxedo-cut jackets and kimono-influenced blouses. But the very best look to come out of the 1970s has to be the floor-length hostess gown, perfect for swanning around at a dinner party, whether in your own home or elsewhere. My pal who was born in 1971 told me that her mom summed up the early 1970s perfectly with this one sentence, written in her baby book: "Richard Nixon was president and hot pants were in!"

In 1972, Dianne von Furstenberg introduced her famous wrap dress to the world, a garment that could take the wearer from office to nightclub with ease. Male disco fans flaunted three-piece suits with wide lapels, while female disco fashions were influenced by modern dance wear, including wrap skirts and dresses made of rayon and jersey. These styles were wildly popular until late 1979, when disco (and the clothes that went with it) fell out of fashion with a bang.

THE 1980S

This decade can safely be described as the decade of the accessory. Costume jewelry was everywhere, with bright gold door-knocker earrings and gumball-sized pearls galore. Madonna took the accessory craze to new heights with her rubber bracelets, fishnet gloves, jangly crucifixes, and lacy headbands—influencing an entire generation of women and young girls in the process. Leotards and leg warmers burst out of the dance world and into mainstream fashion with the start of the aerobics craze, bringing leggings and stirrup pants along for the ride. Keds sneakers worn with slouchy socks were popular among teenaged girls who wore them with fluorescent and neon clothes.

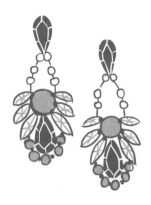

Brand names were hugely important in the 1980s, with Calvin Klein and Ralph Lauren becoming household names by mid-1984. Power dressing meant scores of working women were suiting up, making sure to pop a pair of ferocious shoulder pads into their slightly boxy blazers while climbing the corporate ladder. The silky "bow blouse" is another distinctly 1980s look that feels perfectly right again now—and will for years to come. (They don't call them "classics" for no reason.)

THE 1990S

This was the first decade to begin actively recycling trends of previous eras, specifically the maxi dresses and tie-dye fashions of the 1970s. Ultra-casual dressing took permanent hold in the 1990s, with jeans, T-shirts, hoodies, and sneakers officially becoming the "uniform of the people." Supermodels Linda Evangelista, Christy Turlington, and Naomi Campbell dominated the early part of the decade and set trends—until newcomer Kate Moss ushered in the "heroin chic" and "size-zero fashion" looks in the mid 1990s with her lank, waifish frame.

The rise of grunge music from artists like Nirvana and Pearl Jam made flannel shirts and combat boots one of the hottest trends of the era, culminating in designer Marc Jacobs's famous "grunge collection" for Perry Ellis in 1992. Hip-hop and rap music spawned a proliferation of lifestyle brands focusing on classic streetwear, such as Enyce, Mecca, FUBU, and Lugz.

Slip dresses—whether designer or straight from the lingerie department—were a staple look of the 1990s. Leopard, camouflage, and daisy prints ruled women's fashion, while men's styles veered from Harley Davidson T-shirts worn with wallet chains to overalls with one strap hanging down. Brands like Benetton, Guess, and Girbaud were a must-have for teens of the era—and pieces from all three labels still pop up in thrift stores periodically.

Actress Alicia Silverstone and costume designer Mona May are both responsible for injecting a bit of rich-girl style into the 1990s with the 1995 film *Clueless*. A true homage to teen Beverly Hills fashions of the era (such as matching plaid mini-skirt suits, fluffy angora sweaters, and knee socks), *Clueless* forever made it okay to dress like a prima donna and still be considered cool.

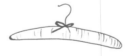

Not only does knowing a bit about fashion through the decades help you spot both real and reproduction pieces in the wild, it's also useful information to have at your fingertips when trying to pinpoint your signature style like we talked about in chapter 4. Otherwise, how would you ever know that you're really a 1950s honey at heart—but with a 1920s twist? When you know what you're looking for (instead of looking for just anything), vintage and thrift shopping suddenly gets a whole lot easier.

But clothing isn't the only thing worth buying secondhand. I happen to think that bags and accessories are the real steal at thrift and vintage stores—so I always keep an eye out for fun scarves, zany purses, and colorful costume jewelry. If you are frowning at this suggestion because your ears are sensitive to cheap metal, it probably means you have a nickel allergy. So do what I do for my actors—clean all earring posts with rubbing alcohol and paint them with clear nail polish before wearing, making sure to allow it to dry thoroughly before inserting into your ears. This creates an invisible barrier between the cheap-o metal and your tender ear flesh, cutting out irritation. You'll have to reapply every so often, but it really does work!

Shopping off-season is also a surefire way to score major deals at thrift stores. It's the law of supply and demand—nobody in their right mind is looking for a winter coat in the middle of July, so it stands to reason that prices will be lower and options more plentiful. And don't ever be afraid to go out on a limb and try something new when buying second hand, whether it's an unusual pattern or a color you've never considered wearing before. The great thing about shopping for used clothing in this day and age is that almost all contemporary clothing is inspired by something vintage—so you actually have a pretty good shot at finding a piece that looks like it could be from a current designer collection. Seek out pieces that are different, unique, and special. If it tickles your fancy, go ahead and try it on! I love using thrift stores as a resource for things I wouldn't normally consider wearing, because the plethora of options forces me to open my mind and gets me out of the "trendy" trap that is so easy to fall into.

ALSO, HAVE A PLAN OF ATTACK

Choose a spot off the beaten path. Thrift and vintage stores in ultra-hip, popular areas are going to be picked over and probably overpriced to boot. The farther outside of a major city you get, the more the prices dive and the more selection there is. Once you're there, don't spend more than an hour in the store. Choose three sections to focus on (such as dresses, pants, and shoes) and give yourself twenty minutes to spend in each. This helps fight fatigue and also gives you ample time to properly examine everything instead of just glossing over an entire rack in a confused daze. You'll then have an additional twenty minutes to try everything on and edit your selections at the very end.

Before you even step foot in a store, be sure to check the going price for various vintage and resale pieces from online vendors so you'll know if you're getting a steal—or just plain ripped off. This will also help you determine if there is any wiggle room in an item's cost—and if a polite inquiry with a sales clerk may yield a lower price. This works best at small, private charity shops—as most major thrift stores have pricing that's set in stone, so asking is likely futile. However, never underestimate the power of a friendly smile and a courteous disposition—as a former retail clerk myself, sometimes that's all I needed to give a customer a small courtesy discount as allowed by my employer. As in life, a little kindness while shopping can go a very long way.

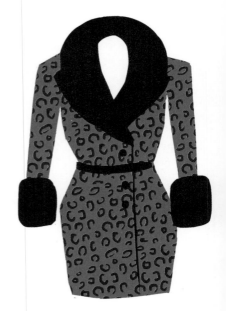

BE SURE TO TRY IT ALL ON
(AND CHECK IT TWICE!)

Yes, you really do have to try it all on. Thrift and vintage stores are pretty much no return affairs—and there's nothing worse than spending money on something just to drag it home and find out that it doesn't fit, then having to relegate it to your own donation pile. This is why it's important to wear something that makes trying on clothes easier. (I like to wear something fitted that acts as a "second skin" so I can basically be nude in public and try everything on even in the middle of the store.)

If trying everything on is your own personal nightmare, I've got the perfect solution: know your measurements. Size tags are notoriously erroneous (and many secondhand pieces have been washed so many times that they've shrunk down considerably from their original size), so I only go by measurements when shopping for an actor. While knowing your measurements sounds like something only movie stars would have access to, it's really not. Having a friend help you figure out your basic measurements is actually quite easy—and keeping them on hand in your bag (along with a small tape measure) while thrift or vintage shopping can help cut the number of garments you actually need to try on in half. The basic measurements you need in order to have an idea of whether or not a garment will fit you are your shoulders, bust, waist, hips, and inseam. (Custom-made garments require a plethora of ridiculously specific details, such as the measurement from your elbow to wrist or neck to belly button, but for the purposes of secondhand shopping, these five will do.)

Armed with your measurements, you can lay most garments flat and measure from seam to seam, doubling the number you get to determine the real circumference of the garment. Numbers don't lie—so if they add up to the measurement you have on the page, chances are it's going to fit perfectly. Here's a handy trick that almost always works to double-check if a pair of pants will fit: take them off the hanger, fasten all buttons and snaps, then wrap the waistband around your neck like a cape. If the seams meet and overlap by about an inch, odds are the pants will fit you nicely in the waist.

One caveat: Ultralow-waisted pants throw this trick off a bit. They don't hit you where your real waist is, so you'll need more fabric overlap (in the neighborhood of three inches) to determine if they will indeed fit. If you're not sure that a particular pair of pants will go over your hips, find the widest part of the pants (through the hip area) and hold them up to your shoulders in front. If the pants are slightly wider than your shoulder span, they will definitely fit over your hips. And you didn't even have to strip down to find out!

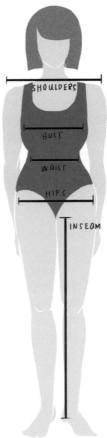

After you've tried everything on, it's time to inspect it all to make sure that it really is in good enough shape to bring it into your closet. Give each piece a serious eyeballing for stains, tears, snags, and pilling. Also, check to ensure that any surface appliques are still intact. Turn the garment inside out and examine it for loose threads along the hem and other hard-to-see issues. Inspect all hardware before buying, such as buttons, zippers, snaps, hook and eyes, or anything else that could wind up needing replacement. Small repairs are fine and even to be expected—but larger issues like tears that aren't along easy-to-fix seams or missing rivets aren't worth the headache unless you are seriously in love with a piece.

Once you've determined that everything you want to buy fits properly and is in good condition, you'll want to do a final "edit" before you hit the cash register. I like to take everything to a quiet part of the store and hang it up, organizing my pieces into yes, no, and maybe piles. A "time-out" from the rush of bargain hunting always helps me make better, smarter purchases that I'm not sorry about later.

FINALLY, GET READY TO WEAR IT

This will be obvious to some but maybe not to others: Before you wear your newfound treasures, you need to wash them. Certain items may need the full professional dry-cleaning treatment—but most of the time, you can apply one of the hand-washing techniques we went over in chapter 10. Just because something doesn't reek of grandma perfume or have obvious stains doesn't mean it's not filthy. A quick soak in the sink will likely make you realize just how gruesomely dirty thrift-store garments can be—so skip this step at your own peril.

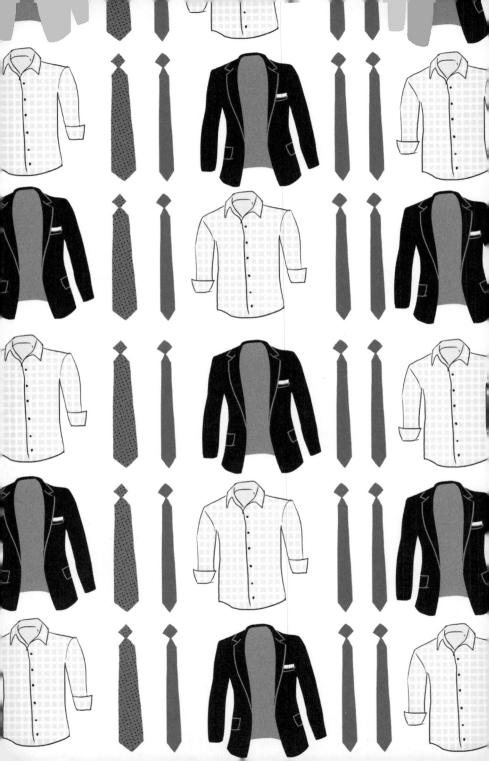

CHAPTER 13

DUDES,
this one's for you

While the person I care most about helping with this book is you, the fact remains that you are eventually going to be faced with having to assist at least one of the dudes in your life with getting his sartorial act together. When that time comes, you can just cut these pages out, pass them over, and consider your work done. But that doesn't mean you shouldn't peek over his shoulder while he reads—because having a working knowledge of men's clothing and style challenges will come in mega-handy when your boyfriend/brother/clueless coworker suddenly needs to look sharp for a major life event (or if you want to dabble in rocking some menswear yourself)! I love dressing male actors simply because men's clothes have so many rules. While the rules for women's fashions are kind of dumb and were made for some serious breaking, classic menswear is all about angles and geometry—so it's a foolproof, mathematical equation that adds up perfectly almost every single time. So much of fashion is pure, glorious, disorganized chaos—but there's a sort of sweet relief in having one single area where order, logic, and strict adherence to style formulas rule the roost.

The cornerstone of proper men's fashion is the humble suit, and wearing one is also the thing that throws most guys for a loop—especially if they are the type of dude who only wears them to weddings, funerals, and job interviews. Awards season in Hollywood is the thing that always stumps the men I dress—suits and tuxedos are the very last thing most guys would usually reach for in their closets. But before you get to playing celebrity stylist, let's discuss how men's clothing is actually meant to fit in the first place. Because as you know by now, proper fit is important. And if something doesn't fit right, it's never going to be stylish.

IF THE JACKET'S NOT RIGHT, THE WHOLE THING IS WRONG

The humble jacket (also known as a blazer) is probably the most important part of a man's look—and a good-looking jacket starts with the shoulders. Remember in chapter 2 when I said that any garment with a poorly fitted shoulder is best avoided? Well, I'm saying it again here. The shoulder is the foundation all else is built on, and if it's wrong, nothing about a jacket is ever going to be right.

A well-fitted shoulder will lay perfectly flat. The seam on top of the shoulder should be the same length as the shoulder bone underneath it and should meet the sleeve of the suit right where the arm meets the shoulder. If the point where the sleeve connects to the jacket is hiked up on the shoulder bone, the jacket won't sit properly. A jacket with a bad shoulder fit will cause an endless amount of lumps, bumps, and wrinkles on the sleeve and at the top of the jacket that no amount of tailoring or alterations can solve.

It's also important to check how the front of a jacket closes over the body. For a single-breasted jacket, close either the top or middle button—even if it's a three-button jacket. The jacket should then meet neatly without the lapels hanging too far forward, which would indicate that it is too loose. If buttoning the jacket causes it to flare out at the bottom, this means the jacket is likely too tight. The buttons should close easily, and there should be no wrinkles beneath the closure. The area below the button should never pull so far apart so as to expose a triangle of shirt above the trousers when standing still. (But when dancing, all bets are off!)

A good sleeve-length guideline for the relationship between a jacket and the shirt worn under it is to always have about a half inch of shirt cuff visible beyond the jacket cuff. Keep in mind, this is only a guideline—styles change with fashion all the time. The only hard-and-fast rule when it comes to sleeve length is that the jacket should never hide the entirety of the shirt cuff. At least a tiny band of sleeve should always be visible. This means that the jacket sleeve will usually end just above the wrist bone. But when in doubt, remember: Flashing a half inch of sleeve will never be considered "wrong."

The ideal length jacket should fall past the waist and drape over the top of the curve formed by the backside, with the hem of the jacket hitting at right about the middle of a cupped hand. If a jacket is sitting on the very top of the butt, creating a small flare in back, it's too short. If a jacket covers the backside entirely, it's too long.

It's quite easy to tell a properly fitting jacket collar from a bad one. For starters, a jacket collar should rest against the shirt collar with no gaps in between. Any space between the shirt and jacket means the collar is too big. A too-tight jacket collar will be a littler harder to diagnose—it will only show itself at the back of the jacket. You'll notice bunching and folds just beneath the collar if it's too tight, and it will often cause wrinkles on the shirt collar as well. A bad collar fit could be the result of a neck size that's wrong for you, but more often than not, it's a sign of a much larger fit issue—such as the dreaded bad shoulder.

THIS IS HOW PANTS SHOULD FIT

The backside (also known as the seat) of a pair of trousers should hang in a smooth drape over the rear end, without pulling tight across it or draping too loosely down the thighs. A bad seat will cause either horizontal wrinkles just under the bum (too tight) or sagging at the backs of the thighs (too loose). A tailor can take in the seat some-what, but there's a limit to how much he or she can do. If the seat is ultraloose, the fit can't be adjusted too far without pulling the pockets out of place. And unless there's a rather large amount of extra cloth in the seat seam of your pants, they can't be let out very far to make a tight pair looser. So when buying a pair of pants, remember: Better to have them a bit too loose than at all too tight.

The break of a pair of pants is the small wrinkle that appears where the top of a shoe cuts into the trouser hem. It should be a small, subtle feature—one single, horizontal dimple is perfect. The pant leg should rest on the top of the shoe, but shouldn't slouch down much farther. Most better dress pants (and almost all suit pants) are sold unhemmed so they can be hemmed to the best length for the wearer.

LET'S TALK ABOUT SHIRTS

A good fit rule for the collar of a shirt is to ensure that only one finger fits comfortably between the collar and neck. If two can fit, it's a sure sign that the collar is too big.

The shirt body poses a special fit issue. Oftentimes, a shirt that fits across the shoulders will be so billowy at the back and torso that you'd think the wearer was hiding a backpack under there. Finding a slimmer cut shirt that also fits through the shoulder area is no small feat— but a shirt that is far too blousy through the body does the wearer zero favors. Persevere until you find the fit that works best for you. Also, the shoulder seams of a well-fitted shirt should hug the shoulders—and shirt cuffs should reach just past the wrists.

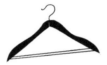

Now you know how basic men's garments are supposed to fit—but you might not have a clue how to determine your correct size. Don't fret, because knowing one's measurements isn't a luxury reserved only for fancy people. Anyone with a tape measure, pen, and a little bit of patience can measure themselves the exact same way a costume designer would—and look far better in their clothes as a result.

HOW TO MEASURE YOURSELF PROPERLY

The measuring guidelines below are most useful when looking to buy a suit or dress shirt and slacks, but having your measurements at the ready is invaluable, no matter what the goal of your shopping trip.

CHEST

Suit and sport coat sizes consist of one number and one letter:
38S, 40R, or 42L, etc. The number corresponds to the chest measurement, while the descriptive letter (which, means short, medium,
or long) refers to the length of the jacket—which is based on height.
Start out by wrapping a cloth tape measure under your armpits around
the fullest part of your chest, making sure the tape is fully crossed over
the shoulder blades in back. The tape measure should be snug—not
so snug as to constrict your breathing, but not so loose that it slides
down. And don't hold your breath, as your chest will then be unnaturally puffed out. The resulting number is the first part of your suit size—
and will likely be anywhere from about 36 to 56. If you are between five
feet four inches and five feet six inches, you are a Short. A height of five
feet seven inches to five feet eleven inches means you're a Regular. And
anyone six feet or over is most definitely a Long.

The waist measurement of the pants that come standard with an
off-the-rack suit will correspond to your jacket size by going down
six inches. This means that if your jacket is a size 40, the pants that
accompany it will have a thirty-four-inch waist. Obviously this formula
doesn't work for all body types, and men who have a greater or lesser
measurement difference will be far better off looking for suit manufacturers who offer separates.

NECK

To buy a dress shirt, you'll need to know both your neck and sleeve
measurements. To determine your neck size, grab the tape measure
and wrap it around the lowest part of your neck, about an inch below
your Adam's apple. Take care not to choke yourself with the tape
measure—for a comfortable fit, you'll want to be able to fit one finger
between the measuring tape and your your neck. When in doubt,
round up to the next half inch.

SLEEVE

Taking a sleeve measurement properly is a two-person job. You'll want to stand with your arm slightly bent at the elbow and your hand on your hip. Your helper should run the tape measure from the very center back of your neck, across your shoulder and elbow and down to just past your wrist joint. The resulting number will be anywhere between twenty-nine and thirty-nine inches, and once you know this number, you'll be amazed at how much better you suddenly look in a dress shirt.

WAIST

Measuring the waist can be a bit tricky, as many men prefer to wear casual pants down around their hips instead of at their natural waists. While this works for jeans and other casual pants, it doesn't fly when you're being fitted for a pair of dress slacks or trousers. You'll want your real, actual waist measurement—taken at around navel level, making sure to put a finger between your body and the tape measure to ensure your pants don't dig into your flesh uncomfortably. The resulting number is your waist size.

INSEAM

Knowing your inseam measurement will save you the cost and hassle of having every pair of pants you ever own hemmed. To figure out what it is, start by standing with your shoes off and hold the end of a tape measure comfortably at crotch level. You don't want to hold it too low, but you also don't want to cram it too far up either. The resulting number is your inseam measurement, and when coupled with your waist measurement, allows you to try on far fewer pairs of pants to find the one that actually fits properly.

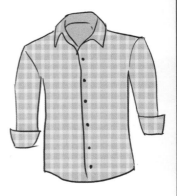

YOU CAN THANK THE DUKE FOR THE SUIT

Now that you know how a suit is meant to fit and how to measure yourself for one properly, how about delving into a little bit of the history of this amazing garment? Because the modern suit really is a miraculous invention. A great suit has the ability to transform even the most slobbish wearer into a creature who at least *appears* to have his life together. The model for modern male elegance in a suit will forever be Edward, Duke of Windsor—also known as Edward VIII, the man who abdicated the throne of England after meeting and falling in love with divorced American Wallis Simpson. The Duke is responsible for establishing innovations in men's suiting fashions during the 1920s and 1930s that remain popular to this day. If you've ever tied a Windsor knot or seen a Windsor collared shirt for sale in a store, you've felt his sartorial influence. Before the Duke, menswear was still stuck in the rigid style parameters of the late 1800s. He cut a debonair figure through the early twentieth century with his easy-cut suits, fresh pattern combinations, and body conscious silhouettes, all of which are now hallmarks of the modern suit.

Looking good in a suit is actually far easier than most guys realize, because a well-cut suit can create an athletic shape where there previously was none, elongate a truncated torso, or camouflage a large belly handily. There's really a suit formula for every single body one could possibly have.

WITH BUTTONS, IT'S SOMETIMES, ALWAYS, NEVER

Once you determine what style of suit to buy, the question of when and how to button it up still remains. The short answer is that suit jackets are meant to be buttoned when standing (to provide a "finished" look) and unbuttoned when sitting so as to keep the fabric from bunching up unflatteringly. Now we've answered the question of when to button, but you're likely wondering which exact buttons you're meant to do up when—and how. Luckily, the art of buttoning isn't all that hard to pick up if you remember three little words: sometimes, always, never. This handy phrase works all the time—whether a suit has one button or three. The top button is your "sometimes" button, with the middle and bottom buttons following as "always" and "never," respectively. This is also a good time to tell you that a suit with more than three buttons isn't a suit—it's an abomination. Never allow any dude in your life to buy or wear one.

On a three-button suit, our "sometimes, always, never" mantra stays intact. On a two-button suit, the top (or "sometimes") button goes away. And on a single button suit, everything except "always" falls away. But one thing never changes: on a suit with two or more buttons, the bottom button is never, ever buttoned up. Legend has it that the custom of leaving one's bottom suit jacket button open grew out of King Edward VIII's ever expanding belly in the late 1800s and early 1900s. The more he ate, the harder it was for him to button up his coat, so he finally did away with buttoning it entirely—and thus, a fashion trend was born. But that was well over one hundred years ago, so you may be wondering why this buttoning rule lasted so long. The reason is simple: it actually does make a suit jacket look better! When you button the last button on a suit jacket, it tends to restrict movement and pull over the hips. It also causes the fabric to bunch up unattractively when you put your hands in your pockets. Leaving the bottom button undone allows the jacket to lay nicely as the body inside the suit goes about its daily business.

I once had a young actor who told me I was dead wrong, and that buttoning one's bottom button was perfectly acceptable. I, of course, politely told him he was incorrect, but he insisted. Rather than argue with him about it at length, I decided to call a comedian pal, who just so happens to be the most dapper man alive and an expert on all things having to do with men's style. I put him on speakerphone with the actor in the room and asked, "Can this young man button the bottom button on his suit jacket in this scene?" To which the comedian casually replied: "It depends. Is he currently standing in a blizzard?"

That was the end of that conversation, and yet another dude in Hollywood now knows the golden rule of suit buttoning by heart.

CAN I TAKE MY JACKET OFF NOW?

Your knowledge of suit etiquette can be determined by how you answer to one single question: When is it acceptable for a man to remove his suit jacket in public?

A: Never.

B: When alone in his personal office, on a plane, or in a car.

C: Whenever he is hot.

D: At a wedding reception.

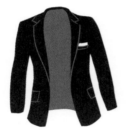 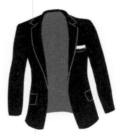

This is a bit of a trick question as the answer is basically A, but also a touch of B. The old-fashioned rule is that a man should never remove his suit jacket when a woman is present, but that should be expanded to say "when other human beings are present." This rule still applies in all business settings and for occasions of any formality. (Yes, this includes wedding receptions and business lunches.) You can obviously remove your jacket when traveling in a plane or car—and in your own office when you are the only one present, it is perfectly acceptable to remove your jacket while you work and hang it on the back of the chair.

But the moment someone enters your office, best practices demand you pop your jacket back on if you want to be taken seriously.

Having said all this, I do believe there is a point in every wedding celebration where debauchery takes hold and removing one's jacket becomes perfectly acceptable. (Hint: It's usually a few hours and a few champagne bottles past 1:00 a.m.) A good rule of thumb is that if the bride's parents have left the building and more than five women have removed their shoes, you're probably in the clear to lose the jacket and dance with sweaty abandon. Until then, keep your suit jacket on tight. If you find that you are uncomfortably hot, it means your suit is made of the wrong material for the weather. Look for seersucker or tropical-weight wools for summertime suit-wearing scenarios.

WHOOPS, THIS SUIT DOESN'T FIT!

Let's say you already own a suit but don't often get a chance to wear it—and as a result, it either doesn't fit anymore or you think it might be a little outdated. You're probably wondering if having it altered is worth it, or if all hope is lost. The correct answer depends on many factors, but the main one is the condition of the suit. If the fabric has become shiny in any area or the cuffs, belt loops, or lining are worn, don't bother. You'll be throwing money away by attempting to tailor it.

As far as fit goes, the most a suit can be altered is to accommodate about twenty pounds in either direction. After that, there are limitations to what can be done to let out or take in a suit before it starts to get proportionally awkward. Two inches from a waistband and about the same around the trunk of a jacket is about the max you can expect to fiddle with a suit before it goes out of alignment and looks bad. And if the shoulders of the suit no longer fit properly, it's time to say goodbye. Lastly (but most importantly) attempting to make a double-breasted suit into a single-breasted suit is wasted money, and you can't make a pair of pleated pants into flat fronts. I've had some success having my tailor stitch down the very top of the pleats on a pair of

HOW TO GET DRESSED

pants to cut down on the "balloon" factor, but it sometimes looks awkward and is best saved for a suit that otherwise has nothing wrong with it. It also works better on cotton suits (like seersucker), since the entire vibe of such a suit is inherently more casual than a wool one.

HOW TO FIX YOUR SEE-THROUGH SHIRT

While it's true that the higher the quality of a dress shirt, the less likely it is to be see-through, sometimes even the most costly shirts can leave a little too much showing for polite company. Luckily, this problem is easily solved by wearing a simple, short-sleeved, crew-necked cotton undershirt. An undershirt also helps keep the front of your dress shirt smooth and tucked in, as the friction between the shirt and undershirt keeps things nice and even. But you may be wondering: "What about when I take my jacket off and you can see my short undershirt sleeves through my dress shirt?" Well, you're not taking your jacket off unless you are traveling or alone, remember? So it doesn't really matter that you can see your undershirt sleeves—because you are the only one who is ever going to see them.

HOW A TIE SHOULD LOOK

While there are endless ways one could tie a tie, I believe there's only one knot you really need to know: the four-in-hand. This is the classic knot favored by businessmen, schoolboys, and lawyers the world over. The size of the four-in-hand knot is on the smaller side, making it ideal for button down and narrow-set collars, although its exact size is dependent on the thickness of the tie's material. The four-in-hand is the epitome of simplicity and style, and if you learn how to tie only one knot, this is it. (It's actually the only one I know how to tie without fear, and I taught myself how to tie it on an actor while in a moving car using instructions I pulled up on my phone!) It will never fail you as it works well with most ties and almost all types of shirt collar. It's also the knot James Bond uses—need I say more?

If you are faced with a shirt that has a wide "spread" (which is the space in between the collar blades), you're going to need to know how to tie a fuller knot to fill in that space—such as the Duke of Windsor's namesake Windsor knot. (I can't ever tie one properly without having to consult the Internet each time, so don't feel bad about not knowing how to tie one already.) The Windsor is the bulkiest knot there is, and the best thing about it is that it stays in place without slipping. A larger knot also has a tendency to draw attention away from the face, so the Windsor looks best on those with a strong jaw or copious amounts of facial hair, as it then helps to strike the proper proportional balance.

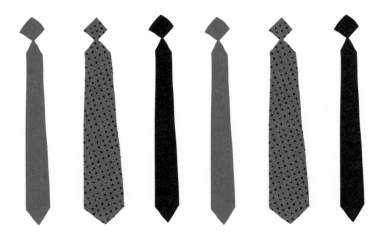

HOW TO WEAR A TUXEDO

Every man will have to wear a tuxedo at least once in his life, even if it's just to the high school prom. Wearing one isn't as daunting as it seems, because a tuxedo is essentially just a really fancy suit. While patterned cummerbunds to match your date's dress are de rigueur for teenagers, wearing a tuxedo as an adult calls for a different set of rules. Even a rental tux can have a bit of savoir faire, if you just know what to ask for. I am of the opinion that if you are going to wear a tuxedo, you're going to want to go all the way. For this reason, opt for a peaked lapel or slim-cut shawl collar. A notch lapel (as found on most business suits) is far too casual.

The number of buttons your tux has depends on your build—just like a regular suit. A two-button tux is a perennial classic, but the fit of a three button style on a taller, broader-shouldered man cannot be underestimated—it creates a flattering "V" shape where a two-button suit tends to gap and pull through the armpits. What's "hip" and what happens to "fit" are two entirely different things, and both should be taken into account when looking for the right tuxedo.

Even if you're stuck with a rental tux, there are still small things you can do to make it look a little richer, a little custom, and a little more special. I like to look for tuxedos that have ribbed silk faille trim on the lapels and pant legs instead of smooth, shiny satin. It's what couture tuxedo-makers like Prada use, and it's an easy way to get a richer, classic look on a cheaper tux.

While the jacket and pants are technically the most important parts of a tuxedo, the shirt you wear matters, too. You want a 100 percent cotton tux shirt, not a thin polyester one. Buying your own slightly higher-quality tuxedo shirt instead of making do with a rental will cost you about fifty bucks and is a great cheat to hide a lesser-quality tux. I like a classic fold-down collar shirt in place of the somewhat dated 1980s-style wing collar, and the good thing about it is that you can then choose to wear either a simple straight or bow tie. But beware: While a fold-down collared shirt looks good with any tux, a bow tie looks best with a peak lapel tuxedo, and a straight tie suits a long, lean shawl collar tux perfectly.

If you choose to wear a bow tie, another good cheat to make your whole getup look more expensive is to spring for a real, old-fashioned, hand-tied bow tie. Make sure you buy one that matches the trim on your tuxedo's lapel and pants leg, and have someone at the store tie it for you, making sure to keep two fingers under the band to ensure it's tied somewhat loosely on the neck. You can then carefully snip the tie at the back of the neck and take it to a tailor, asking them to stitch down the bow in front and add a strip of Velcro or a hook at the back so you can easily put it on just like an adjustable one. While this might seem like a ridiculous amount of work, nothing kills a formal look faster than an adjustable metal clip showing anywhere on your tie band. The Velcro cheat is one we use on any show that calls for a bow tie, as hand-tying one is a skill that not even many costumers have.

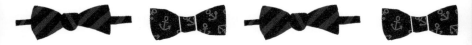

But what about cumberbunds? While patterned or brightly colored ones are indeed a hallmark of the prom-style tuxedo look and have no place on a grown adult, that doesn't mean you can do away with one entirely. The rules of tuxedo wearing dictate that you must have something to hide the awkward transition between the shirt's edge and the workings of the trousers' waistband. Letting this seam fly free and uncovered is akin to a woman walking out of the bathroom with her skirt tucked into her underwear and her panties flapping in the breeze. A tux worn without the waistband covered is an incomplete look and a grave fashion faux pas. If you opt for the classic cummerbund look, wear it pleats up and make sure it matches the fabrication of your tie, which then in turn matches the lapels of your jacket and the trim of your pants. If a cummerbund isn't your speed, you can opt to wear a vest (either full-backed or cutaway) to cover your waistband instead. But if you think wearing a vest then gives you license to remove your jacket in public, you are dead wrong.

I know exactly what you're thinking after reading all this nonsense about waist covering: "But I see movie stars on the red carpet not wearing a cummerbund all the time!" There is some truth to this statement, but let's separate a little fact from fiction here. Almost without fail, the stars working this uncovered waistband look have tux pants that are specially designed with a slightly wider satin-covered waistband as a stand-in for a cummerbund. Secondly, their outfits have been chosen with only one purpose in mind—standing on the red carpet and having their photo taken. And even with their jackets closed, these stars still sometimes have a bit of unflattering white shirt peeking out when they put their hands in their pockets, causing the jacket to spread apart. Pulling this same look off in real life is quite the challenge. Rules in formal wear exist for a reason, and if you want to be taken seriously, it's worth taking the time to learn them. (Or at least be aware of them so you know when you are breaking them.)

As if we didn't talk about buttons enough earlier in this chapter, let's have a few more words about them now. Some fashion purists still insist that leaving your shirt buttons exposed on a tuxedo shirt is up there with showing your waistband on the list of tux-wearing "no-nos." The truth of the matter is that exposed shirt buttons are actually perfectly acceptable in this day and age. But, if you want to go old-school, you have two choices to solve this problem: either choose a shirt with a covered button placket or get yourself a set of button covers.

If you choose to go the button cover route, I like the look of simple white satin ones so they blend in with the shirt. When a stark white shirt (unfettered by distracting plastic buttons) is set off by a beautiful hand-tied bow tie and a proper waist covering, everything but a man's face and personality falls away, allowing both to shine. And that's the real reason for rules in suiting and formal wear—to let the man in the suit be front and center, without a lot of faddish, complicated clothing choices mucking up the works.

Unless you are attending an incredibly formal event at the request of a European monarch, you can do away with the dated, old-style patent leather tux shoe. I much prefer a cap- or rounded-toe dress shoe done up in super-shiny smooth leather. As for the somewhat recent trend of wearing sneakers with a tuxedo to a wedding, they are no more appropriate there than they would be at a court appearance. The point of a tuxedo is to dress up for once in your miserable life, so go ahead and wear a pair of big-boy shoes for a few hours, would ya?

Go Ahead, Sit on the Grass: Stain Glossary

Unless otherwise noted, always lay your freshly treated items on a clean, dry towel and allow them to air-dry completely so you can determine if the stain is indeed fully removed. If you get too zealous and pop the item in the dryer before checking to see that stain is really gone, you'll likely have set the stain in for life. You'll also notice that in some cases, I recommend using paper towels for initial stain blotting, but quickly move on to using a clean white cloth. Paper towels break down easily when excess pressure is applied, and little rolled-up bits of frayed paper towel are the last thing you need in the mix when attempting to remove a stubborn stain.

ASH (CIGARETTE)

You'll need: liquid dishwashing detergent and two clean white cloths.

+ Mix one tablespoon of liquid dishwashing detergent with two cups of cool water.

+ Using a clean white cloth, dab the stain with the detergent solution.

+ Blot with a dry cloth until the garment is damp, not wet. Repeat until the stain disappears.

+ Rinse garment and launder immediately. (If garment is not machine washable, spot clean the affected area with diluted liquid laundry detergent and take it to the dry cleaner as soon as possible.)

BEER

You'll need: liquid dishwashing detergent, white vinegar, rubbing alcohol, a clean sponge, and a clean white cloth.

+ Soak the garment for fifteen minutes in a mixture of one-quart lukewarm water, one-half teaspoon liquid dishwashing detergent, and one tablespoon white vinegar.

+ Using a clean sponge, dab at any remaining stain with rubbing alcohol, working from the center to the edge of the stain. Blot with a dry cloth to determine progress.

+ Rinse garment and launder immediately.

BLOOD

If you don't care to lick your bloodstains away, you'll need: a blunt kitchen knife, liquid dishwashing detergent, ammonia, and a clean white cloth.

+ Scrape off any excess material with a blunt kitchen knife.

+ Soak the garment for fifteen minutes in a mixture of one-quart lukewarm water, one-half teaspoon liquid dishwashing detergent, and one tablespoon ammonia.

+ Remove the garment from soaking without rinsing and blot the stain gently from the back with the clean white cloth to loosen. (This is key—blotting from behind helps push the stain forward and out of the garment's fibers.)

+ If stain has been removed completely, rinse garment and launder immediately.

+ If the stain remains, give the item another fifteen-minute soak in the same water-detergent-ammonia mixture. Repeat the blotting from behind, rinse well, and launder the garment only when the stain is fully removed.

CANDLE WAX

You'll need: ice cubes, dull kitchen knife, an iron, and paper grocery sacks or paper towels.

+ Rub wax stain well with ice to "freeze" residue. Carefully scrape off as much material as possible with a dull kitchen knife.

+ Place a paper grocery sack or folded paper towels both over and under the

wax-stained area and gently press with a warm—not hot—dry iron. Do not use steam.

+ Wax will begin to melt and be absorbed into the paper bag or towel. Repeat with clean paper materials until no more wax remains. Check and change the paper frequently—it is quite easy to accidentally reintroduce wax residue onto the garment by reusing paper that has previously absorbed wax.

+ Launder the garment only if all wax residue has been removed.

CHOCOLATE

You'll need: a blunt kitchen knife, liquid dishwashing detergent, paper towels, and a clean white cloth.

+ Scrape any excess material off with a blunt kitchen knife. Blot the stain with a paper towel to remove any additional surface material.

+ Place paper towels under the stain and saturate the area with liquid dishwashing detergent. Allow to penetrate for one minute and then blot from the top with more paper towels or a clean white cloth.

+ Rinse, launder, or hand wash immediately.

COFFEE

You'll need: liquid dishwashing detergent, white vinegar, rubbing alcohol, and a clean sponge.

+ Soak the coffee-stained garment for fifteen minutes in a mixture of one-quart lukewarm water, one-half teaspoon liquid dishwashing detergent, and one tablespoon white vinegar. Remove from solution and rinse thoroughly.

+ Using a clean sponge, dab at any remaining stain with rubbing alcohol, using light motions from the center to the edge of the stain.

+ Rinse garment and launder immediately.

COLA

You'll need: white vinegar, liquid laundry detergent, 3 percent hydrogen peroxide, paper towels, a spray bottle, and a clean white cloth.

+ Blot stained area with a paper towel to remove as much cola as possible, then saturate stain with a white vinegar solution (one-third cup white vinegar in two-thirds cup of water). Using a spray bottle filled with plain, cold water, work at the stain, blotting with more paper towels to remove excess moisture.

+ If stain persists, apply a small quantity of detergent-peroxide solution to the spot. (To make the solution, mix one-quarter teaspoon liquid laundry detergent with one quart of water, adding two capfuls of hydrogen peroxide.) Using a clean white cloth, blot the stain carefully to work the detergent-peroxide solution into the affected area. If stain is being removed, continue applying solution and blotting until stain is completely gone.

+ Rinse garment and launder immediately.

GRASS

You'll need: an enzyme-based stain removal product (like Zout Triple Enzyme Clean Formula.)

+ Soak the grass-stained garment in a solution of cool water and a product containing enzymes for at least thirty minutes—or overnight for aged stains. (This gives the enzymes time to digest your stain.) Do not use hot water; it will coagulate the proteins in your enzyme-based stain removal product and make the grass stain more difficult to remove.

+ Rinse garment and launder immediately. Avoid using hot water as it can set the vegetable dye in grass stains.

+ If stain still remains, soak an additional thirty minutes in fresh solution and re-wash immediately.

INK

The old wives tale is that hair spray removes ink. This used to be absolutely true back when hair spray had a higher alcohol content, but today's hair sprays are sadly lacking—to remove an ink stain, you'll need: rubbing alcohol, a clean sponge, and a clean towel.

+ Flush the stain with ice cold water, making sure to work from the back of the stain.

+ Next, place the stained garment on a clean, dry towel and use a clean sponge to work a small amount of rubbing alcohol into the stain, again working from the back. The stain should begin to leech out onto the towel.

+ Rinse garment and launder immediately to remove residual ink.

KETCHUP

You'll need: liquid laundry detergent and an enzyme-based stain remover.

+ Pretreat by applying liquid laundry detergent directly to the stain.

+ Do not allow liquid laundry detergent to sit on the garment; dyes in detergent can stain when applied in undiluted amounts. Rinse, launder, or hand wash immediately.

+ If the stain persists, move on to treating the area with an enzyme-based stain remover; then rinse, launder, or hand wash immediately.

+ If stain still remains, and your garment is white (and 100 percent cotton), you can try soaking it in a heavily diluted solution of liquid chlorine bleach and warm water. A good rule of thumb is to use no more than three capfuls of bleach to one gallon of water. Chlorine bleach can rapidly change the color of a garment and cause irreversible damage (including yellowing of white garments), so check for bleach tolerance on a hidden seam. If stain does not come out within fifteen minutes of bleaching, it cannot be removed by bleaching. Do not allow garment to soak for longer than fifteen minutes, as fibers will start to break down. Rinse garment and launder immediately after treating.

MAKE-UP (OIL BASED)

You'll need: liquid dishwashing detergent, paper towels, and some waterless mechanic's soap (such as Mechanic's Friend, commonly used in auto garages to clean up oil spills.)

+ Remove excess makeup by blotting with paper towels. Then, saturate area with liquid dishwashing detergent. Allow detergent to sit for fifteen minutes, blotting dry with more paper towels.

+ Rinse garment and launder immediately.

+ If stain remains, repeat process using waterless mechanic's soap in place of liquid dishwashing detergent.

MAKE-UP (WATER BASED)

You'll need: liquid dishwashing detergent, white vinegar, rubbing alcohol, and a clean sponge. (For plain white, 100 percent cotton garments only, you can use diluted liquid chlorine bleach—but remember, no more than three capfuls of bleach per gallon of water!)

+ Soak the garment for fifteen minutes in a mixture of one-quart lukewarm water, one-half teaspoon liquid hand dishwashing detergent, and one tablespoon white vinegar.

+ Rinse garment and launder immediately.

+ If makeup residue remains, work carefully at the stain using a clean sponge and rubbing alcohol with light motions from the center to the edge of the stain.

+ If stain still persists, launder garment in cool water with a capful of liquid chlorine bleach (if fabric allows.) Otherwise, use two capfuls of color-safe oxygen bleach in a cool wash load.

NAIL POLISH

You'll need: ice, dull kitchen knife, nail polish remover or acetone, and paper towels.

+ Allow nail polish to dry completely before attempting removal.

+ Rub dried polish with ice to "freeze" residue and carefully scrape off as much excess material as possible with dull kitchen knife.

+ Apply nail polish remover or acetone to the back of the stain, protecting the front of garment with a pad of paper towels or other absorbent material. Do not apply nail polish remover to any synthetic fabric, which it will cause the material to melt. This process works best on cotton, linen, denim and wool.

+ Rinse garment and launder immediately.

SALAD DRESSING (OLIVE OIL)

You'll need: baking soda, cornstarch or another absorbent powder, liquid laundry detergent, and paper towels.

+ Gently blot the stain with paper towels to absorb as much surface material as possible.

+ Sprinkle powder on stain, allowing it to sit on the garment's surface for five minutes. Gently blow the powder off the stained area—don't brush, as it can inadvertently grind the stain in.

+ Pretreat stain by applying liquid laundry detergent directly to the stain. (Do not allow liquid laundry detergent to sit on the garment; dyes in detergent can stain when applied in undiluted amounts.)

+ Launder garment immediately.

WINE

You'll need: liquid dishwashing detergent, white vinegar, rubbing alcohol, an enzyme-based stain removal product, and a clean sponge.

+ Soak stained garment for fifteen minutes in a mixture of one-quart lukewarm water, one-half teaspoon liquid dishwashing detergent, and one tablespoon white vinegar.

+ Carefully blot stain with a clean sponge using a solution of rubbing alcohol diluted with water. Use light motions from the center to the edge of the stain. (Alternatively, you can soak the garment in a solution of cool water and enzyme-based stain removal product for thirty minutes or more.)

+ Rinse garment and launder immediately.

Take Care of What You've Got:
Fabric Care Glossary

Figuring out how to take care of your clothes properly can be a real head-scratcher when you don't even know what you're dealing with in the first place. The handy fabric glossary below covers most everything you're likely to have in your closet—and is a great resource to consult before you do something to a garment that could damage it irreparably.

ACETATE

A chemically engineered, silky textured fabric made from plant matter, usually wood pulp. Commonly used in linings of coats and dresses; it is lightweight and soft against the skin. Take great care when washing as acetate can shrink and wrinkle very easily. Because of this, it is best sent to dry cleaner.

ACRYLIC

An artificial textile made from petroleum products, first developed by DuPont in 1950. Usually has a knitted appearance and often used in sweaters, but is not as warm as wool. Resists moth holes, stains, fading, and wrinkling handily. Wash in warm water in your machine or by hand, using fabric softener. A few drops of fabric softener will help fight static cling, something acrylic is known for. Dry at low temperatures because acrylic can melt or scorch easily.

ANGORA

Made from the downy coat of the Angora rabbit. Smooth and silky, it is incredibly warm and often used for sweaters. Many retailers have stopped selling Angora products due to concerns over animal cruelty as rabbits are often plucked. A rest in a humid room such as a bathroom will cause wrinkles to fall out easily. Hand wash and air dry according to methods outlined in chapter 10.

BAMBOO

A soft, natural fiber that is naturally bacteria and odor resistant, as well as super absorbent and breathable. Makes great socks, underwear, and casual clothing. Machine washable and dryer safe.

BATIK

A traditional Indonesian fabric originally created using a wax-resistant dyeing technique. Melted wax is applied to the fabric before it is dipped in dye, resulting in intricate patterns wherever the dye cannot penetrate. Real batik pieces are usually rendered in cotton or silk, and great care should be taken when washing them to protect the dye from running. Hand washing with very cold water and ultragentle detergent is a must, and a color-catching cloth (like the Shout Color Catcher sheet) will help trap and absorb loose dye in the wash water.

BOUCLÉ

Wool bouclé (French for "curled") is a classic nubby fabric created by wrapping at least two different yarns into a twisted pattern. Bouclé is popularly used in women's suiting, most notably in styles from the House of Chanel. As almost all suiting pieces are lined, bouclé should be professionally dry-cleaned.

BROCADE

A thick, loom-woven fabric that is usually shot through with gold or silver threads and has a raised pattern. The classic Chinese cheongsam is an example of a brocade garment. Brocade was historically loomed using silk fibers, but most modern-day brocade is of synthetic origin. Silk brocades can be carefully hand washed, but synthetic brocade has a tendency to unravel when agitated, so dry cleaning is safest.

BURNOUT VELVET

Created when fiber-eating chemicals are painted on velvet fabric. A sheer, negative space remains as a pattern. Usually made of silk or synthetic. Unlike regular velvet, burnout has a very short pile, so treat it

as you would any other silk or synthetic fabric, by careful hand washing or dry cleaning.

CAMEL HAIR

A thick, warm, luxury material, similar to cashmere. Made from the underwool of the camel. Extremely soft. Usually found in overcoats. Dry-clean lined camel hair jackets for best results.

CANVAS

An extremely heavy-duty, plain woven fabric often used for sails, backpacks, and sneakers. Usually made from cotton or linen. Can stand up to heavy use and repeated high-temperature washing and drying.

CASHMERE

A very warm, lightweight, natural fabric woven from the soft undercoat of the cashmere goat. Prone to pilling due to fibers rubbing together during wear, which can easily be removed with a fabric shaver or disposable razor. Hand wash and air dry according to methods outlined in chapter 10, adding a bit of fabric softener to help fibers retain elasticity.

CHAMBRAY

Chambray originated in the town of Chambrai in northern France and is woven from cotton or synthetic fibers. Usually made using blue and white yarns, chambray has a pale, frosted, denim-like appearance. Machine washable and dryer safe.

CHARMEUSE

A silky fabric with a shiny face and dull back, similar to satin but lighter weight. Usually rayon, but sometimes made of silk. Often used in blouses and cocktail dresses. Hand wash and air dry unlined charmeuse garments according to methods outlined in chapter 10.

CHIFFON

A lightweight silk fabric that is extremely sheer and has a slightly rough texture. Unless intricate pleating or folds are present, hand wash and air dry according to methods outlined in chapter 10. Chiffon snags easily and needs diligent, gentle pressing to retain its shape. For these reasons, you may prefer to dry clean.

CORDUROY

A ribbed, cotton-blend fabric that is very warm and quite sturdy. The ribs are called "wales" and range in thickness from three to twenty-one ribs per inch. Machine washable and dryer safe

COTTON

A sturdy, natural fiber derived from the cotton plant. Breathable, machine washable, and endlessly comfortable.

CREPE DE CHINE

A heavy satin fabric that has the crinkled texture of crepe on one side, while the other has a smooth, shiny finish. Often used for formal gowns, as it drapes and hangs beautifully. Best dry-cleaned to protect color and sheen.

DAMASK

A heavy, usually self-patterned woven fabric made from either cotton, linen, silk, or wool and commonly used for draperies and upholstery. Damask's woven texture is prone to unraveling, so hand washing, gentle cycle laundering, or dry cleaning is a must.

DENIM

A heavyweight, hardworking, twill cotton weave fabric made with two different colored yarns to produce its signature blue shade. Premium denim should be washed in cold water inside out and air dried to prevent shrinking and fading, but most denim is machine washable and dryer safe.

DOUBLE KNIT

A double-thick constructed fabric created by two layers of fabric being woven together. Very flattering and smoothing. Can be made of wool, cotton, or polyester. Sometimes has added stretch. Most unlined double knits can be washed in cool water and hung to air dry. Resists wrinkles. Great for traveling.

DUPIONI SILK

A silk fabric that does not separate the worm's cocoon during the weaving process, creating a slub texture in the fabric. Often used in women's separates. If colorfast, okay to hand wash as outlined in chapter 10.

FAUX FUR

Made of synthetic fibers, usually petroleum based, and meant to resemble real fur. Fake fur can be spot cleaned using a baby wipe or "dry cleaned" with cornmeal. Sprinkle a healthy amount of dry, ground cornmeal onto soiled areas, first laying down plastic to catch excess. Work cornmeal into fabric well and allow to sit for several hours. The cornmeal will absorb oil, dirt, and grime. Take garment outdoors and shake vigorously to remove excess cornmeal. Brush carefully with a slicker brush (commonly used to groom cats) to fluff up matted areas and remove any lingering cornmeal. If grime persists, machine wash fake fur pieces inside out in very cold water on delicate cycle using gentle laundry soap, adding a small amount of liquid fabric softener to rinse cycle. Hang to dry and fluff "fur" with slicker brush if necessary.

FELT

A dense, matted wool fabric created by rolling or pressing wool fibers with water or heat. Hand wash and air dry as outlined in chapter 10, taking great care to reform felt to original shape after washing, gently stretching if needed to avoid shrinkage.

GABARDINE

A tightly woven fabric historically made of wool that resists wrinkling. For the shopper on a budget, polyester gabardine is a good stand-in for wool. Commonly used in suits and slacks. If unlined, gabardine can be hand washed and air dried according to instructions outlined in chapter 10. But fair warning: Wool takes forever and a day to dry.

GAZAR

A somewhat stiff silk fabric that is slightly sheer and has a faint sheen. It folds and drapes beautifully and is often used in wedding gowns. Gazar is one of the few silks that should be exclusively dry cleaned to retain its shape. Not to be confused with organza, a silk fabric that is more sheer.

GEORGETTE

An airy, lightweight, twisted silk fabric that has a crinkled "broomstick" texture. Georgette feels slightly rough and dull but has a bouncy, flowing look. Can be hand washed and air dried according to instructions outlined in chapter 10.

JERSEY

A cotton knit fabric that usually has a small amount of stretch. Commonly used to make T-shirts, jersey can be machine-washed and tumble dried on low safely. Finer-spun jersey is made of rayon and has a slinkier hand, suitable for dresses, skirts, and tops. Rayon jersey can be hand washed and air dried according to instructions outlined in chapter 10. Rayon jersey is non-wrinkling and excellent for travel.

LAMÉ

A fabric made by the weaving together of thin ribbons of metallic yarn made of nylon or polyester. Often used for theatrical costumes or evening wear, lamé threads have a tendency to pull and slip, resulting in frayed areas over time. Lamé is best dry cleaned to maintain shape and prevent "tarnishing" of metallic fibers.

LINEN

A loose-weave, breathable, durable fabric derived from the flax plant, suitable for very hot climates. Prone to excessive wrinkling, but responds well to either machine or hand washing and air drying. Give linen a quick pressing while still damp to help retain shape. Lined linen pieces should be dry cleaned to ensure lining does not shrink or warp.

LUREX

A name-brand, synthetic fabric made of metallic yarn, which consists of polyester and a vaporized layer of aluminum. As with any metallic fiber, Lurex should be dry cleaned as infrequently as possible and never ironed.

MERINO WOOL

An exceptionally soft, warm, thin, fine wool that does not itch or scratch when worn close to the skin. Can be hand washed and air dried according to instructions outlined in chapter 10. Too-frequent dry cleaning can dry out and damage merino wool.

MICROFIBER

A synthetic polyester-based stretchy fiber that is far thinner than a strand of human hair. Commonly used in sweat-wicking workout garments and shapewear. Machine wash and air dry to maintain elasticity, as excessive heat is the enemy of stretch materials.

NYLON

A generic tern for any synthetic fabric made of thermoplastic. Used in slips, sportswear, windbreakers, and track pants. Nylon can be machine washed and tumble dried on medium heat without fear. Nylon melts if exposed to high tem-peratures.

ORGANZA

A thin, sheer, crisp, open-weave silk fabric similar to gazar, yet far more sheer. Commonly used for wedding garments and petticoats. Organza is best dry-cleaned to retain shape and crispness.

PEAU DE SOIE

Dyeable wedding shoes are often made of peau de soie, a heavy-ish weight silken polyester fabric that takes dye evenly and completely. Peau de soie shoes can be carefully hand or machine washed by placing them in a pillowcase for protec-tion and allowing to air dry.

POLYESTER

A category of polymer-based fabrics known for their durability, wrinkle-resistant properties, and long wear. Polyester can be safely machine washed and dried on medium heat, but will scorch at high temperatures.

RAMIE

One of the world's oldest fibers, ramie is a natural fabric made from the China grass crop. It is resistant to mildew, stains, and insect attacks, and launders like a dream in cool or warm water. For best results, machine wash and hang ramie garments to dry (wrinkles will fall out) and store flat. Ramie fibers can be brittle and prone to breaking when left hanging.

RAYON

Rayon is a manufactured fiber created from regenerated cellulose, also known as wood pulp. As with acetate, rayon has a tendency to shrink and weaken when wet. Hand wash in cool water and lay flat to dry or dry clean infrequently for best results. If pressing is needed, use a warm iron on the wrong side of garment while still damp.

SATIN

Often used in evening and formal dresses. A heavyweight silk fabric with a glossy, smooth surface and dull back. Hand wash inside out in cool water and allow to air dry for best results.

SEERSUCKER

A thin, puckered, all-cotton fabric commonly used for summer suiting. Usually striped or checkered, with a slight wrinkled appearance. Most seersucker suiting is lined with cotton and can therefore be hand washed and air dried easily. Press seersucker garments carefully to remove large wrinkles yet retain its rumpled charm.

SHARKSKIN

Commonly used in men's vintage-style suiting and usually made with either acetate or rayon. Sharkskin is created by weaving two different colored threads on the diagonal with pure white fibers. This results in a two-toned, iridescent "sheen" that changes colors depending on the light. Acetate and rayon shrink rapidly when exposed to water, so sharkskin should always be professionally dry cleaned.

SILK

A strong, lustrous fabric produced by harvesting the cocoon of the silk moth caterpillar. Do not fear hand washing silk; it is a protein fiber—just like hair. Treat your silk garments as you would your hair, and you'll be fine. Hand wash and air dry silk according to the directions in chapter 10. Do not soak longer than 10 minutes, and never spray deodorant or perfume on silk. Silk is prone to perspiration stains, so consider using armpit guards as discussed on pages 82–83.

SPANDEX

A durable, expandable, synthetic fiber with great elasticity, commonly used in swimsuits, bras, leggings, and exercisewear. Lycra is a brand-name version of spandex, often used in better control undergarments. Lycra and spandex can be machine washed in warm water—and air dries in minutes. Exercise wear made of spandex can tend to hold odors, but a presoak of one cup white vinegar to one gallon cold water for thirty minutes followed by a warm wash will usually eradicate all funk. Never use fabric softener on spandex, as it can build up and leave a coating on garments.

SUITING

A finely woven, high-quality wool fabric meant for suits, trousers, jackets, and skirts. Suiting pieces are almost always lined and most jackets contain an inner layer of fused fabric or canvas, rendering them dry clean only. Too-frequent dry cleaning can lead to a rough, orange peel texture at a suit jacket's front. To avoid this phenomenon, wear armpit guards as discussed on pages 82–83 to keep sweat stains at bay and hang suiting pieces in an area where air can move freely through them to freshen up between wearings.

TAFFETA

Taffeta is a crisp, smooth, woven fabric made of rayon. Often used in wedding gowns, bridesmaid dresses, and curtains, rayon has a lustrous, glimmering appearance. Rayon taffeta can lose its crisp texture when exposed to water, so professional dry cleaning is preferable.

TULLE

A very fine, lightweight netting, which is often starched. Used for veils, ballet tutus, and as embellishment on evening gowns. Tulle tears easily and should always be hand washed. Never put tulle in the dryer; exposure to heat can melt the material.

TWEED

Tweed is a rough, unfinished, woolen fabric, suitable for informal outerwear due to its moisture resistance and durability. Tweed has been produced for centuries in Scotland and Ireland. It can be carefully hand washed and laid flat to dry as long as there is no lining present. Take the time to reshape freshly washed tweed garments before they dry to prevent shrinkage and never, ever put tweed in the dryer.

ULTRASUEDE

Ultrasuede is a brand-name, microfiber fabric meant to be a substitute for suede leather. It has a slight raised nap and lends itself to jackets, sport coats, handbags, and pants. Ultrasuede resists wrinkling, is ultraeasy to care for, and can be machine washed and hung to dry.

VELOUR

A synthetic, plush, knitted fabric with a nap similar to velvet. Often used for casual and leisurewear, velour can be machine washed and tumble dried on medium. Resists wrinkling and pilling. Creases in velour can be removed by light steaming.

VELVET/VELVETEEN

Velvet is a plush fabric with a heavy pile and a brilliant sheen. Real velvet is made of silk and should be dry cleaned as infrequently as possible, as both water and excess chemicals can damage its luster. Velveteen is imitation velvet, often made of cotton, and is safe to machine wash and dry on medium heat.

VISCOSE

Viscose is a form of rayon fabric that can be machine washed on the gentle cycle in cool water. Viscose becomes weak when wet, so care should be taken not to stretch or stress fibers unnecessarily. Air drying is best.

VOILE

A soft, thin, sheer fabric meant for summerwear, usually made of cotton or polyester. Most voile is preshrunk, making it machine washable. Low heat or air drying is best to prevent shrinkage. Never use chlorine bleach on voile, as it can rapidly eat through thin fibers.

WOOL/VIRGIN WOOL

Virgin wool is simply wool that has not had any processing to remove its natural oils. As a result, it retains some moisture-repellant properties and warmth. Often used for sweaters and socks, virgin wool can usually be hand washed and laid flat to dry, taking care to reshape the garment while still wet. However, wool that has been treated with a finish should be professionally dry cleaned only, as washing can result in shrinkage. Wool items with lining or shoulder pads should never be washed. Protect your wool clothing from moth damage by shaking out and brushing wool pieces periodically, making sure they are clean before storing, as moths are attracted to body oils. Cedar and mothballs are only effective against moths when their odor is quite strong. Wearing an undershirt beneath wool pieces cuts down on the need for laundering and most stains can be removed with a stiff bristle brush. Pills on wool can safely be dispersed using a fabric shaver or disposable razor.

Acknowledgments

I would be absolutely nowhere without the support of my family: my dad Doug, my mom Jackie, my brother Paul, and my love Tommy Blacha. Tommy always told me when what I'd written was good—but also pointed out how it could be better. And from the very first conversation I had with Kaitlin Ketchum, my editor at Ten Speed, I knew she was the one for me. Her combination of super smarts and perfect skin has never steered me wrong. I'm also forever grateful to my English and journalism teachers at Round Rock High School in Round Rock, Texas—Mrs. Spencer and Mrs. Komandosky, who taught me how to write. I heard their words in my head whenever I was stuck.

I owe many, many thanks to all the local 705 costumers who covered for me on set while I hunched over my laptop in the corners of endless wardrobe trailers, writing while the cameras were rolling. I'm also very blessed to have some seriously talented pals: Chad Kultgen, Chuck Hayward, Laurie Parres, James Merrill, and Tara Touzie—your encouragement, laughs, insights, and jokes are what got me to the finish line.

I'm incredibly grateful to Holly Schmidt and Becky Thomas for convincing me to write a book in the first place—and to Ten Speed designer Margaux Keres and illustrator Julia Kuo for bringing my words to life with incredible style. Also, thank goodness for Jane Pratt and Emily McCombs at xoJane.com, who took a wild chance on a weirdo who only ever wanted to write about clothes. But absolutely none of this fairy tale would have happened without Bianca Dorso and Steve Rice telling me that I could be a costume designer all those many years ago—and then believing in me until it happened.

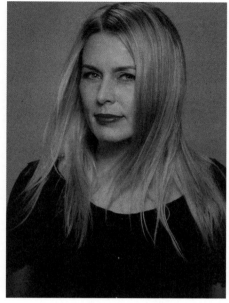

Olivia Malone

About the Author

Alison Freer is a costume designer from Texas, living in Los Angeles, California. She dresses people for television shows, commercials, music videos, and films. This means she shops every single day and has turned numerous inanimate objects into wearable costumes. In her spare time, Alison writes about fashion, clothes, and style on xoJane.com as the resident clothes editor. She doesn't believe there are any "rules" for fashion, and neither should you.

Index

A

Acetate, 225
Acrylic, 225
Alterations
finding tailor for, 42–44
importance of, 30–32, 46, 98
"instant," 76–77
with poor return, 40–42
for suits, 211–12
terms for, 44–46
worthwhile, 32–39
Angora, 225
Armpit stains, 82–83, 148
Ash stains, 219

B

Bamboo, 225
Batik, 225–26
Beer stains, 219
Belt hole punch, 82
Belts
color of, 62
storing, 103, 107, 111
Topstick and, 79, 80
Bike shorts, 119
Blazers. See Jackets
Blisters, 182
Blondes, wearing yellow, 69–70
Bloodstains, 158, 220
Blouses
altering, 33–34, 36–37
proper-fitting, 21–22
Boots
short, 64
storing, 110–11
in the summer, 64
Bouclé, 226
Bow ties, 214–15
Bras
with backless garments, 138–39
finding right, 124, 129–35

going without, 123–24, 139
putting on, 133
sizes of, 130–32, 133–34
storing, 106–7
styles of, 124–29
tweaking existing, 81, 135–39
washing, 140
Brocade, 226
Bunions, 182–83
Burnout velvet, 226
Buttons
keeping closed, 76
on men's suits, 208–10

C

Camel hair, 226
Camisoles, 95–96, 111
Candle wax stains, 220
Canvas, 226
Cashmere, 226
Chambray, 226
Charity shops, 186
Charmeuse, 227
Chiffon, 41, 227
Chocolate stains, 220
Cigarette stains, 219
Clothing
dyeing, 164–65
inappropriate, 95–96
quality vs. quantity of, 98–99
sizing of, 30–31
storing, 102–14
See also Fit; Laundry;
Menswear; Vintage and
used clothing; individual
clothing items
Coffee stains, 220–21
Cola stains, 221
Colors, choosing, 61–63, 65–66, 68–70
Consignment shops, 187
Corduroy, 227

Costume designers
role of, ix–x, xii
for TV shows, 8–9
See also Wardrobe fittings
Cotton, 227. See also individual
cotton fabrics
Crepe de chine, 227
Cumberbunds, 215–16

D

Damask, 227
Darning, 46
Darts, 36, 45
Denim, 67–68, 227. See also
Jeans
Double knit, 227
Dresses
altering, 34–36
proper-fitting, 24–27
strapless, 26, 75
styles of, 24–27
zippers on, 85–87
Dry-cleaning, 152–57
Dyeing, 164–65, 178

F

Fabric care, 225–32
Felt, 228
Fit
concept of, 12–13
style and, 12, 27
See also Alterations;
individual clothing items
Flip-flops, 76
Fur, faux, 228

G

Gabardine, 228
Garment bags, 112–13
Gazar, 228
Georgette, 228
Granny panties, 119
Grass stains, 221

Published in the United States by Ten Speed Press, an imprint of the
Crown Publishing Group, a division of Random House LLC, a Penguin
Random House Company, New York.
www.crownpublishing.com
www.tenspeed.com

Ten Speed Press and the Ten Speed Press colophon are registered
trademarks of Random House LLC.

Library of Congress Cataloging-in-Publication Data

Freer, Alison.
How to get dressed / Alison Freer.
     pages cm
1. Clothing and dress—Handbooks, manuals, etc.
2. Fashion—Handbooks, manuals, etc. I. Title.
TT515.F74 2015
646'.3—dc23
                          2014036765

Trade Paperback ISBN: 978-1-60774-706-2
eBook ISBN: 978-1-60774-707-9

Printed in China

Design by Margaux Keres

10 9 8 7 6 5

First Edition